Food intolerance and how to deal with it

Delicious plant-based recipes with juicing ideas

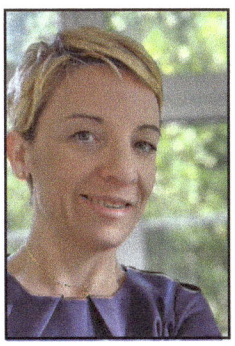

Kinga Krisztina Lőrincz

Published by Dolman Scott in 2025

Copyright©2025 Kinga Krisztina Lőrincz

All rights reserved. No part of this publication may be reproduced, stored in a retrieval system, or transmitted in any form or by any means, electronic, mechanical, photocopy, recording or otherwise, without prior written permission of the copyright owner. Nor can it be circulated in any form of binding or cover other than that in which it is published and without similar condition including this condition being imposed on a subsequent purchaser.

ISBN: 978-1-915351-44-9

Published by
DolmanScott
www.dolmanscott.com

To my loved ones…

"The power of our God was with us and protected us.

Paul writes, "What great persecutions I have endured, and the Lord has saved me from them all!

Someone always helps me when I lose my courage.

This is He, who knows me and loves me and restore my strength daily—He is always with me." (Bible)

Contents

Introduction 1

Food sensitivity or intolerance 2

Symptoms and solutions.. 4

Scientific presentation of the digestive system in a nutshell..... 8

Conclusions... 12

The scientific perspective on the relationship between stress
and food intolerance 18
    1.   What is stress? 18
    2.   How stress is related to digestion................................. 18
    3.   How stress triggers intestinal hypersensitivity.......... 20
    4.   Gut bacteria and stress 20

Superfoods... 22

Favorite recipes 29

Summary 59

Inspired by... 61

Introduction

Welcome to everyone who is reading this book. You have likely decided to do so because you have some interest in your own health, the health of your family or your friends. This is not unusual, as many of us who find ourselves in these situations start researching, trying to find answers to questions for which doctors do not always know the solution, unfortunately. Such problems can range on a scale from mild to terrible. In my own experience, I turned from the emergency room further to a specialist, from the general practitioner to various procedures. I knocked on several doors and found different answers, but I did not recover; in the meantime, I also became exhausted by the way in which I was treated. Even though I was seriously ill, it was very difficult to find a compassionate specialist. Also, it seemed strange how little was known about my symptoms, and I am not exaggerating when I say that I couldn't find a doctor who could not only give me advice but heal me. At one point I even believed there was no chance of recovery from this "unknown disease". After a while, when I was already weakened and couldn't find a way out, I decided that it would be better to start researching my "problem" myself, as I didn't know anything about food intolerance, its causes or its various manifestations. I am going to tell you about my own story, in the hope that you may recognize yourself and the different states I have experienced, in which case, this book will be of help to you. The purpose of the book is not to give medical advice, but to disseminate knowledge and curiosity. It's very important to understand that if someone is seriously ill, they should first seek advice from their own doctor, before considering other alternatives.

Food sensitivity or intolerance

In the case of food intolerance, the body's system is unable to digest food because it lacks sufficient enzymes. However, there may be other reasons for this, and symptoms can appear a few hours or even days later. Food intolerance is different from food allergies, which are caused by an abnormal response from the immune system. This occurs when the immune system mistakenly recognizes a food ingredient as dangerous – usually proteins – and triggers defense reactions against it, in which case the symptoms appear immediately and can range from mild to severe, or even fatal. Furthermore, they can also be confused with the symptoms of other diseases. The question that crossed my mind is: how do we know what makes us sick and how do we decode the various symptoms our bodies use to signal that there is a problem? It's true that our bodies are very clever at sending us signals when something extraordinary happens to our body, but do we pay enough attention to them? Various questions may arise in our minds, when we're in pain, should we go to the doctor immediately or should we wait a little longer? We find ourselves at a crossroads with a decision to make, but we need to remember that our health is not a trivial matter; it's always worth going to the doctor as soon as we notice a problem. But what if we keep going to the doctor, but we still never find a solution to the problem? When I reached this point, I began researching to find my own answers. I was not aware of how and why I had become sick; all I knew was that it was not the result of an injury and it was not due to an accident. I was not imagining it either; I was experiencing a genuine illness. I'm sure you've been there—you've explained all your symptoms, the different kinds of pain, your thoughts about it all—only to be treated as though you're making it up. But don't be intimidated. Keep your head up.

I didn't have the time or energy to get angry when I got reactions like that; I used what little strength I had left to get stuck into my own researching.

Symptoms and solutions

In Medias Res … cut to the chase, long story in short, this experience not only changed my health, but the way I got to see the world, the gratitude, the happiness, the compassion I feel, makes a difference. My symptoms were very different from the beginning. First, I made notes when they appeared, so that I could compare any changes later. Symptoms are the messages of our body, even so they can be painful, the body is powerful, and this power is working for you. Eventually, I had experienced all of the following symptoms: nausea, loss of appetite, bloating, headache, inflammation in the body, pain in the bones, continuous inflammation of the ear, nose and throat, abdominal cramps, low blood pressure, widespread pain, lethargy and excessive fatigue, anxiety, dizziness, brain fog, reflux, very dry mouth, rash (mainly on the back), and a lot of sudden infections. My ill health reached a particular low point when I was infected with the COVID-19 virus, when I almost lost my life due to blood poisoning. Much later, I discovered that some of the food I liked to eat so much, didn't like me back. For a while, I didn't want to accept this. Psychologically, I felt broken, but I was still strong enough to continue further with my research.

It did not take long for me to understand the reason for my despair, the absurdity I found myself in. Should I look for the cause or rather the solution to the problem at all? I continued searching for the truth.

Complicated questions were buzzing around my head, as I wondered where I might find the solution. Eventually, the thought came to me: Was it likely to be an external factor, an internal factor or a combination of these that had made me sick? If it was caused by external factors, how did these manifest themselves, and if it was an internal cause, how did it encounter my body?

That's how I reached the point of realizing that whatever we put in our mouths eventually comes in contact with our organs and can therefore be the cause of health problems—not to mention the side effects of various medical treatments and the prolonged use of antibiotics, which is often not helpful for our bodies. What is the point of eating? Many people don't understand this. Is it a question of love or a question of existence? Food is a tool, a propellant, a nourishment for the body; it is a force that drives us physically, but it is definitely not the meaning of life. The meaning of life lies not in what we eat, but in being together with our families and loved ones, going out and enjoying nature, and rejoicing in the beautiful sunshine and our closeness to God!

By putting it into a philosophical framework, and rejecting all other ideas, I put into practice the little information I had gathered from my studies, and—in tiny but purposeful steps—I set out on the path of science, which brought success. You might think that it was easy, but it wasn't. I was facing a long, bumpy road, but my heart was full of trust and faith. The following words from the Bible were next to me: "Our God is strong"; this made sense in my head immediately and I saw a light at the end of a narrow tunnel. I followed it devoutly, because I felt that I was on the right path when my research met my "reality". By putting it into practice, I was able to build on what I had already known by adding my newly discovered facts. The results brought a new feeling I had been longing for; that of being healthy! This new feeling of freedom had me shouting for joy as I achieved small successes at the cost of great sacrifices.

A lot of people in the world die every day due to various addictions, including drugs, alcohol, and medicine. Actually, the number one killer in America is heart attack in people says Dr. Brook Goldner (2025). Statistics have shown that poor dietary choices are a leading cause of death. Such choices include processed food, packed with preservatives, which may be tasty but not healthy, others contain an awful lot of animal products; these allow for the further accumulation of toxins in the liver and elsewhere in the body. Most people eat meat several times a day, without even thinking about the animal cruelty involved. In fact, they would not starve to death without meat, but they eat it anyway for pure enjoyment. People have developed an addiction to food they don't know anything about; their eating choices are formed from habit, following patterns and beliefs they've absorbed unquestioningly since birth. Everyone seemed surprised when I talked about this. Not only did they not understand, but some even found it unacceptable. When it comes to food, illogical, unthinking people will eat whatever they want; they will not give up their favorite food, even in the face of a heart operation, kidney failure, or excessive weight gain. If they are asked: why they say: "I love the food", they will answer that they love to eat, but that most of the time the food doesn't love them back—they seem amazed by this! And yet it is no wonder that they then suffer from various autoimmune diseases, digestive disorders, fatty liver disease, diabetes, kidney failure, high cholesterol levels, heart problems, pancreatic cancers, arthritis, osteoporosis and so on. The root cause is impermeable bowel syndrome, and all of them have one thing in common: inflammation in the body, which can be completely eliminated with a proper diet and lifestyle. This is what I did, and how I achieved my physical recovery. Making a list of all the foods I ate every day, I then eliminated all the foods I couldn't eat. Based on my research, I started to use the elimination diet. A lot of foods were soon removed from the list. I was left with a shortlist that grew even shorter, consisting mainly of fruits, vegetables, gluten-free products, chia seeds, lentils, and vegetable milks, including coconut milk, oat milk, and rice milk, as well as rice and corn grits. In addition to this, I took vitamins A/B complex/ C/ D3 and K/E/ probiotics/ iron/and minerals separately. I was sensitive not only to food, but also to vitamins, medicines, creams, and smells, and I could not tolerate loud/sharp sounds or bright light. High levels of histamine started to show up within the symptoms.

At the end of each month, I summarized what I had experienced, the symptoms that had appeared, and those that had ceased. Furthermore, I underwent many blood tests, blood formulas, vitamin/mineral tests, various X-ray tests, allergy tests. I suggest that intolerance tests are not worth doing because scientists have shown these kinds of tests for food intolerance are not reliable. Also, I took a magnetic resonance test and finally a comprehensive stool test, which provides a broad picture of the health of the intestinal flora, including the multitude of "good" and "bad" bacteria, and the presence of parasites and various fungi. The main one is the well-known candida albicanis, which, in my case, was the culprit and needed to be eliminated; if untreated, it would have been a significant obstacle to my further recovery. Candida albicanis is a type of yeast that is a common part of our microbiome but can cause infection when it overgrows. The process of healing from the fungus itself was long, but I later realized that fungi do not have to be "killed" from the body; instead, you need to find the best way to reduce their number, while simultaneously feeding the growth of "good" bacteria in the intestinal flora. Importantly, you need to accept them as part of your functioning body. You got to understand the way they work in your body and finding a way to cooperate with them. There are countless bacteria, parasites, and fungi living in the intestinal flora, and their functions and interactions with each other are vitally important. It is worth paying attention to the intestinal flora and supporting it by reintroducing healthy food into your lifestyle, especially fruits and vegetables.

Continuing my research, I was looking for the underlying cause of the problem when I came across some studies that provide very important information for anyone who has struggled with digestion as I have. During my last visit to the doctor, I was diagnosed with fibromyalgia. Don't be scared by hearing the term fibromyalgia; it is a symptom that comes from a complex of various other diseases, and it is closely related to leaky gut syndrome, but it is also a symptom that many people experience having undergone some form of trauma, depression, emotional/physical abuse, or psychological and psychiatric disorders. Therefore, anyone experiencing this is well advised to seek psychological/psychiatric support as well. In my case, fibromyalgia had a different meaning; it was a physical symptom, manifesting as physical pain and fatigue. My goal was to investigate the root cause of it, which I did.

Scientific presentation of the digestive system in a nutshell

The human digestive system is a complex organ system whose function is not only to digest and absorb food, but also to excrete waste products. It works closely with several other organs and organ systems (central nervous system, liver, bile, stomach, pancreas, small intestine) that are discussed in more detail in this topic. The proper functioning of our body depends on the regulation of our hormones, nervous system, and other organs. Digestion begins in the oral cavity and ends in the rectum. The proper size and physical digestion of the food taken into the oral cavity is ensured by the teeth. The stirring motion and grinding by the tongue allow the food to homogenize, and the food mobilizes the appropriate enzymes. An average of 1-1.5 liters of saliva is produced per day. Saliva is produced by the salivary glands, which include the parotid gland (near the jaw), and the sublingual gland (under the tongue). Saliva itself is composed of both organic and inorganic substances.

1.**Organic:** amylase enzyme that breaks down starch and glycogen. Its function requires calcium and chloride ions, as well as a slightly alkaline pH, so it does not show significant activity in the acidic environment of the stomach.

2.**Inorganic:** at first, the composition of saliva is the same as that of blood plasma. Active and passive ion flows can be observed in the salivary glands and their outlet tubes. Its calcium ion content prevents calcium from escaping from the teeth in a slightly alkaline environment. Due to the secretory activity of the salivary glands, some toxic substances are excreted in saliva. Only a small number of substances is absorbed from the mucous membrane of the oral cavity. The next part that is involved in our digestion is the esophagus. When food enters the oral cavity, it triggers the swallowing reflex, which results in a coordinated movement of the pharynx and esophagus. In the esophagus, saliva retains its functions and from there food travels towards the stomach. In sync with the esophagus, the upper sphincter ring of the stomach opens. Longitudinal and transverse folds can be seen on the gastric mucosa. The fold is capable of autonomous movement, which is made possible by the mucous membrane's own muscle layer. The muscle layers on the walls of the stomach make a stirring-kneading movement, while food is transferred to the outlet part of the stomach. These movements in the stomach wall are coordinated by the autonomic nervous system network. The gastric juice in the stomach fulfills many functions. An adult produces an average of 2.5-3.5 liters of gastric juice per day. Stomach acid activates pepsinogen, which breaks down proteins in the form of pepsin. In the absence of stomach acid and pepsin enzymes, the proteins in the stomach are not broken down. In the stomach, food is mixed with stomach acid and enzymes, which further break down proteins. Unfortunately, many people do not produce enough stomach acid, and what is produced may also be blocked by acid inhibitor pills. Stomach acid is vital for efficient digestion. With the intensive movement of the stomach, the mixture turns into a dense, semi-liquid substance. The acidic environment of the stomach helps not only to break down food, but also to destroy pathogens. Another important stage of digestion involves the small intestine. From the stomach, the digested food is excreted intermittently into the small intestine, where digestion is continued by the bile and pancreatic juices emptied there. The gut flora in the digestive tract, also known as the microbiome, is vital for our health. Gut bacteria not only help break down food, also support the functioning of the immune system. Research shows that a healthy gut flora contributes to improved mood and better mental well-being. Bile is produced by liver cells, before being stored or condensed in the gallbladder. The bile acids in the bile emulsify the fat, making it water-soluble, thus activating fat-breaking enzymes. It does not contain bile enzymes. Bile acids are compounds formed from cholesterol. Only 5-10% of the bile acids that enter the small intestine are excreted in the feces, with the rest being reabsorbed and recirculated. Bile also contains bile dyes, cholesterol, lecithin, proteins and other organic metabolites. The main stimulus for the excretion of bile is the entry of fats into the small intestine. Pancreatic juice is the exocrine secretion of the gland. The outlet tube of the pancreas, together with the bile, enters the small intestine. The pancreas only begins to secrete the sap during eating. The main stimulus for this is the ingress of acidic stomach contents into the stomach, as a result of which the pancreas produces alkaline enzyme-free juice, which neutralizes the acidic stomach contents, thus providing the right conditions for the enzymes. Generally, inactive enzymes are produced in the pancreas and become active in the intestinal tract, thus avoiding the self-digestion of the organ. Carbohydrate breakdown is continued by amylase produced in the pancreas, then fat breakdown is carried out by lipase, and its activation is due to calcium and bile acids. The next stage takes place in the following sections of the small intestine: fasting intestine (ileum), iliac intestine (jejunum) 8-20 liters of small intestine juice are produced daily; this contains protein-degrading, carbohydrate-degrading (amylase, sucrase, maltase, lactase) and lipid-degrading (lipase) enzymes. Its most important task is to absorb nutrients, which are thus broken down into the basic units that enter the body. From here, nutrients move into the large intestine, including the appendix, ascending colon, transverse colon, descending colon, and sigmoid colon. Although often overlooked, the large intestine does play a role in digestion, primarily through fermentation and putrefaction. In the initial half of the colon, ferments producing acidic products predominate, while in the other half in an alkaline medium, protein decomposition processes dominate. This will produce partially toxic, foul-smelling compounds. Finally, the digestion process ends in the large intestine, where water and minerals are absorbed and the remaining substances are excreted from the body. The bacteria in the colon help break down residual nutrients and form stool. **The link between digestion and mental health is increasingly becoming the focus of scientific research. The so-called gut-brain axis represents the communication network**

between the gut and the brain. Compounds produced by gut bacteria, such as serotonin, have a direct effect on brain function and mood. A study from the Mayo Clinic has shown that a healthy gut flora and proper digestion can help reduce the symptoms of depression and anxiety. The production of various vitamins is carried out by the non-pathogenic intestinal bacteria present here. These bacteria obtain energy from undigested carbohydrates through a fermentation process, and the final products are used by the epidermis covering the inner wall of the intestine. In addition, water and electrolytes are absorbed, especially in the initial stages of the colon. The stool collects and is stored in the sigmoid intestine until it reaches the right amount and is transmitted to the rectum, where digestion ends. The process of digestion is not just about breaking down food and absorbing nutrients. This complex system plays a fundamental role in maintaining our health and mental well-being.

Conclusions

When we begin to experience success, our motivation to continue what we have started increases.

The relationship between food and humans should never be an estrangement; instead, there should be a direct, open and fair relationship between the two. It is important to recognize when food is not working in harmony with your body, and to summon willpower to leave it out of your diet. When food goes on your plate, it prepares to become part of your own body and blood. Therefore, we must respect the food we eat, as it's set to become part of our own bodies. Our body responds positively to what gives it life—but it can rebel against anything that hinders its growth and well-being. We should nourish ourselves with natural foods, the way nature intended; they are gifts of the earth that support health and balance. Once, I asked someone what his diet looked like and what medical issues he was struggling with. He said that he suffered with his thyroid gland and was not sick because of food. But what if the food he ate didn't serve his body, didn't support his digestive system, or was even causing his thyroid disease without his knowledge? The food we put into our bodies can be medicine, but it can also be poison, depending on whether it is in harmony or disharmony with our body. What is good for one person can be bad for another. Do not look for answers from a whole list of symptoms but consider them individually. I learned not to try to overcome my illnesses, but rather to figure out how my body worked and what imbalances were pushing me in the wrong direction. A very important question to consider is: Are you aware of eating assertively? Nowadays, there are a lot of different diets around. I'm not a fan of diets; they are a waste of time and money. If a doctor prescribes a certain diet for a short time, it must be for a specific reason. That's different from a person throwing themselves into a weight loss diet that he truly believes will work, while depriving his body of food that he will no doubt overcompensate for the following month. Then he will find himself in an even more serious situation, because unfortunately a "diet" will never work; it needs to be a lifestyle change. If someone wants to follow a healthy lifestyle, they should forget about diets. Instead, they should focus on how to create a feasible lifestyle in harmony with their body and follow it continuously. The lifestyle itself encompasses not only the food we eat, but also the quality and quantity of sleep, human relationships, exercise, the workplace, our thoughts, stress levels, and relaxation. All of these are examples of issues that need to be considered in order to keep your body in a healthy balance. We often wonder why we are tired, or what can be causing our back pain. We may wake up several times during the night, and we might find countless excuses to try to explain what the cause might be, but if all this is happening in the long term, it is worth looking for the cause in the digestive system. Our internal organs have created a close connection with each other; if one of them does not work at full capacity, then the task falls to our other organs and hinders not only its ordinary work, but also its ultimate goal of survival, for which our body fights every day. A very good example of this is when not enough stomach acid is produced in the stomach. Stomach acid is needed to break down proteins, primarily under the influence of pepsin and acid, so if there is an insufficient amount then the bile slows down, and the pancreas is not able to produce lipase in the absence of stomach acid and bile acid, which is needed to break up the food that has already reached the stomach into small pieces before sending it to our next organ to process the food. Low pH in the stomach indicates low stomach acid, so no pepsin is released, meaning that the food as a whole is not broken down. Different groups of symptoms indicate a possible problem, such as indigestion and gas in the intestines, stomach cramps, belching, and pain. In this case, the bile is not able to produce enough bile acid, so the pancreas has to compensate for this. If a person has had their gallbladder removed, they are recommended to take bile enzymes during meals, which promote digestion and also support the pancreas. Others may be struggling with stomach bloating and diarrhea, but still have bile, in which case we also have to pay attention to the color of the stool. If it is white or very light brown or yellowish in color, this indicates a lack of bile acid (but at the same time the pancreas is incapable of breaking down fats and protein, as it does not produce lipase either). In this case, it is worth eating bitter foods at this time (artichoke/ beetroot/ginger/ turmeric/ parsley greens/ pepper mustard/radish/asparagus garlic). Bloody swallowwort/lemon balm, dandelion, peppermint/chamomile/ginger/wormwood) and bile enzymes can be consumed (tudca /milk thistle/ ox-bile/ beetflow) to replenish bile acid, which does not digest food. When it reaches the small intestine, it indicates irregularity undigested, with various severe or mild symptoms. I recommend paying attention to prevent such problems. We should strive to treat the root of our diseases, rather than to "patch up" the symptoms, which only helps for a short time. Bile acid can also be measured at home with urine test strips, by measuring bilirubin and urobilinogen.(T.C Hale,2012). The liver uses bilirubin to produce bile acid, which is a fluid that promotes digestion in the small intestine. Its deficiency can be caused by the use of low-fat foods, stress, the use of steroids, and too many carbohydrates in the diet. If someone suffers from stomach pain, bloating and ongoing constipation, it is often due to a lack of stomach acid. You can try a home remedy: mix apple cider vinegar in water and drink it before every meal, or put sea salt in a glass of water, which can be extremely helpful in digestion. If the constipation persists, you can take HCL gastric acid capsules for a while until the need in the stomach is satisfied. However, these should not be used in the case of gastric ulcers. If you suffer from a deficiency of bile acid, it is worth supplementing the bile acid with stomach acid (T.C Hale, 2012). There are several reasons for a lack of stomach acid. First of all, as we get older, less is produced. The lack of electrolytes also affects acid production; the same process happens with different enzymes in our body, so it is worth paying attention to them. If you are struggling with these kinds of problems, it is worth trying these remedies. I recommend taking care to examine the histamine-supporting DAO enzyme; if it has a low level, there is a high probability that a high level of histamine has been produced in the body. We will talk about this in more detail elsewhere. Some people suffer from long-term reflux, which can seriously damage the esophagus in the long term. In this case, the doctor will often prescribe stomach acid blockers as the primary treatment. Over the years, this condition may worsen as, according to the latest statistics, 90% of people suffer from low stomach acid, which can be caused by a lack of minerals, especially zinc and B vitamins. As a result, low blood pressure is also common in such cases. In the absence of stomach acid, bacteria can easily enter through the mouth to the stomach, so it plays a key role in digestion. When we find that we cannot consume certain foods that contain a lot of protein and fats, we should consider the above suggestions, but at the same time, consider the lack of pancreatic enzyme or pancreas functioning, which is the production of lipase and amylase. The pancreas is known for other functions besides the production of enzymes, including the production of hormones, one of the most important of which is insulin. Various blood tests can be used to detect their enzyme value. In terms of deficiencies, we must check which enzymes are missing and replace them with supplements if necessary (I use plant-based supplements). If we do not take action, we could easily find ourselves with food intolerance. Although we may put considerable energy into solving the problem, we may not be able to, as there are often a lot of symptoms that even a doctor is unable to recognize. In this case, take the difficult approach of elimination to identify which foods you cannot consume and forgot them for a month or two. Then reintroduce the foods back into your diet one by one and, if you start to feel unwell, continue to avoid them. Another aspect that we cannot ignore is the leaky gut, which affects the small intestine, where digestion takes place. In connection with the digestive problems listed above, initially we must heal the intestines first. This requires changing our diet, but also our lifestyle, including sleep, as well as dealing with everyday stress, human relationships and exercise. I have only mentioned the most important of these, but do not exclude others; when you recognize an issue as causing a problem, you should do something about it. Leaky gut has not necessarily received formal recognition in gastroenterology. No specialists deal with the treatment of the small intestine, and it does not appear in medical guidelines as a specific medical condition. When I started researching it, I found it to be an abstract concept. An inflammatory health problem, leaky gut is a condition whereby the epithelial cells of the intestinal wall are weakened, allowing foreign substances to enter the blood and thereby triggering inflammation and immune responses. If you are struggling with the following symptoms, it is worth paying attention and treating it before your health deteriorates: abdominal pain, bloating, belching, gas, diarrhea or constipation, sudden weight loss, muscle weakness, anemia, hormonal system breakdown, muscle pain, brain fog, irritability, insomnia, anxiety, depression just to name few of it. The small intestine is the part of our stomach where the most important operations take place; it is the busiest part of our body, where the extraordinary microbiome, "good" and "bad" bacteria, parasites, and fungi live together, contributing to our happiness and health while keeping us alive. It might seem surprising that our digestive system can make us happy! Our digestive system is closely connected to our brain, through the "vagus nerve", which is the largest and most key parasympathetic nerve in our body. It is like the brain of our gut, and its innervation extends to its abdominal organs; it is a motor and sensory nerve, which is called the planetary nerve because from the moment it leaves the skull, it enmeshes the abdominal organs through the neck, which carries information from the body to the brain, so if our digestion is not working, we will encounter many psychological symptoms. These include anxiety, depression, foggy brain, dizziness, insomnia, forgetfulness, and confusion. In the case of leaky gut, we need to support the small intestine with certain products. The following are examples from natural sources I've tried: marshmallow root tea, aloe vera gel, elm tea, probiotics for balancing the intestinal flora (lactobacillus /bifidobacterium / paracasei/ plantarum/ rhamnosus/ acidophilus), spirulina, chlorella, homemade drinks from cruciferous vegetables, green tea, ginger, turmeric, and lemon. Don't forget that healing the body begins from the inside and works its way out. We should not only focus on healing the body, but also the soul. We should not choose a 'diet', but a healthy life, while also letting go not only of what hurts the body, but also of anything harming the soul. Step out of the 'mold' in which you live, be happy with yourself and love yourself.

Don't try to make others happy; this should not be the purpose of your life. Love everything and everyone. Embrace the new and let go of the past. Many of us carry the traumas of the generations in our souls. Each generation has resolved these according to the possibilities afforded by their circumstances; you also solve yours with the tools that are available to you. If you can't do this on your own, consult a specialist.

The scientific perspective on the relationship between stress and food intolerance

What is stress?

We all worry that excessive stress will make us sick. It's important to remember that stress is caused by the way in which we react to the environment; it is not necessarily a reflection of the world around us. Some people do not feel stressed when they are climbing high mountains or speaking in front of thousands of people. On the other hand, others find shopping at the supermarket, driving a car or talking to their boss very stressful. Stress reflects our own response to the environment, not an external stimulus. Stress reactions are a normal part of human existence and help protect us from injury. As humans evolved thousands of years ago, early humans who were anxious to escape predators survived to have more children, whereas their more laid-back counterparts did not! So, a certain degree of stress is normal and part of a healthy life.

How is stress related to digestion?

It is easy to recognize that stress affects the gut. We all get the common symptoms of butterflies in the stomach or have to go to the toilet when we're feeling stressed. But how much worse can it get? How dangerous is the impact of stress on digestion? Many people wonder whether stress can really cause problems such as ulcers, cancer or intestinal inflammation. People with irritable bowel syndrome often recognize that stress is exacerbating their symptoms – so what can be done about it? With normal nausea, abdominal complaints and stress, the urgent need to go to the toilet is due to the close connection between the brain and the intestinal tract. Many types of nerves are shared between the brain and the gut brain, which is called the gut-soluble nervous system. Some people even call this connection the "big brain, small brain" or "gut-brain axis". The two "brains" talk to each other. Sometimes I compare the relationship to that of a small child and a parent; they are often caring and harmonious, and sometimes they can definitely pull each other up! When we get stressed, the body triggers a so-called "fight or flight" response. This has a number of effects, including increased movement in the intestine and a decrease in blood flow, which is diverted to other organs. When the gut becomes stressed—perhaps due to an infection, food intolerance, or bacterial change—it also reacts with a change in movement and sends pain messages to the "big" brain. Symptoms that can occur as a result of stress include the following:

- Increased heartbeat
- Blood vessels constrict
- Increase in blood pressure
- Increase in blood sugar levels
- Increase in respiratory rate
- Sweating increases
- Change in stomach acid levels
- Changes in the contraction of the digestive muscles
- Hormonal imbalance
- Digestive muscles are affected
- Affected gastric secretions
- Changes in enzyme activity
- Changes in intestinal bacteria
- Increased risk of inflammation

Stress can trigger allergic reactions in the gut and other organs, and depression or anxiety can exacerbate the symptoms of inflammatory disorders in the gut.

One of the many challenging tasks of the gastrointestinal tract is to develop an aggressive response to gut-soluble microbes while maintaining tolerance to food antigens and commensal bacteria (The American Journal of Pathology, 2006).

How stress triggers intestinal hypersensitivity

Stress can upset the digestive system. When you're stressed, your nervous system sends signals to your gut and intestines, triggering the digestive muscles to enter into a "fight or flight" response. For example, they may react by pushing waste through the system quickly, causing nausea, cramping, bloating, or diarrhea.

Gut bacteria and stress

Evidence suggests that stress in both animals and humans causes changes in gut bacteria. Studies have also shown that stress changes the bacteria in animals, as well as the bacteria in patients with depression. Good bacteria reduce stress responses in animals, but as yet there is no clear evidence that the same is true for humans. However, there is still much research to be done in this area. Certainly, it is true that diets high in fiber, fruits and vegetables are associated with lower rates of mental illness in adults and adolescents. How can we avoid bowel problems caused by stress? Managing stress often requires examining changes in many aspects of lifestyle, as well as using individual techniques to induce relaxation. In her article, journalist B. Eva Glamour (2024) writes:

"In Andrea Trenja's experience, people underestimate the impact of state of mind on digestion, appetite, or bowel habit. From whether someone has too much or too little stomach acid, how much bile is produced, whether they have an appetite, how fast their digestion is, to when they can pass a stool, all of these are related to their spiritual orientation," the specialist points out.

Superfoods

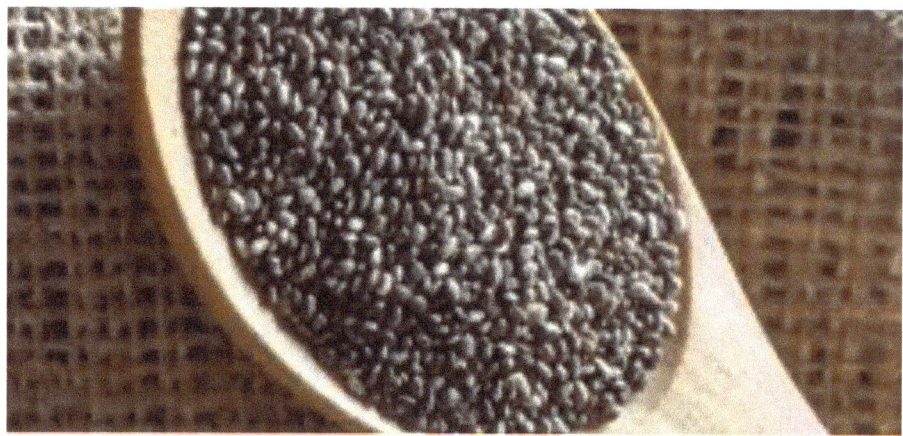

Chia seeds are an important source of polyunsaturated fatty acids, particularly due to their high omega-3 content. Regular consumption of chia seeds may play a significant role in the prevention of heart disease, diabetes, cancer, and depression, as well as contribute effectively to improved blood cholesterol levels. In addition to being rich in unsaturated fatty acids, chia seeds provide substantial dietary fiber, which can benefit digestive health, they also contain considerable amounts of minerals such as magnesium, potassium, selenium, iron, and zinc, all of which support the maintenance of healthy skin and hair. Zinc supports hair and nail nourishment and is involved in cell formation; selenium offers protection against harmful UV rays; iron may help reduce hair loss; and B vitamins stimulate hair growth. Incorporating chia seeds into the diet may therefore be advantageous for those seeking healthier hair and radiant skin. Notably, one of the most significant benefits attributed to chia seeds is their potential to reduce inflammation in the body.

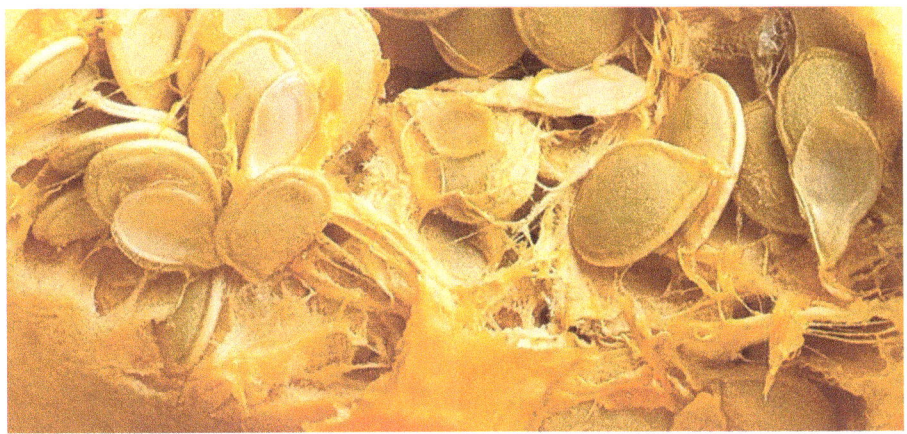

Pumpkin seeds offer numerous health benefits and are easy to add to your diet. They are rich in magnesium, iron, zinc, phosphorus, potassium, antioxidants, fiber, and protein, while being low in fat and calories. These nutrients support heart health, digestion, immune function, and may help lower blood sugar, improve sleep, reduce inflammation, and benefit skin and brain health. Regular consumption can also address issues like prostate problems, insomnia, iron deficiency, and osteoporosis. Pumpkin seeds are high in antioxidants as flavonoids and phenolic acids. They also contain small amounts of vitamin E and carotenoids. Some research suggests that pumpkin seeds may contain plant compounds that could help protect against cancer growth. Pumpkin seeds are one of the best natural sources of magnesium, a mineral that is often lacking in our diets. Pumpkin seeds are controlling blood pressure, reduces heart disease risk, forms and maintain healthy bones, regulates blood sugar levels

Spinach is an annual plant that grows up to 30 cm tall. Spinach can be eaten both cooked and raw. The taste of raw spinach is mild, slightly sour, it fits perfectly in salads, and its vitamin A and C content is significant, although most of the latter is dissolved during cooking. It contains nutrients useful for our body in a concentrated form. Such nutrients include manganese, which acts as antioxidants, copper, zinc, vitamin E and selenium; vitamin B1, vitamin B2, which provide energy, calcium and

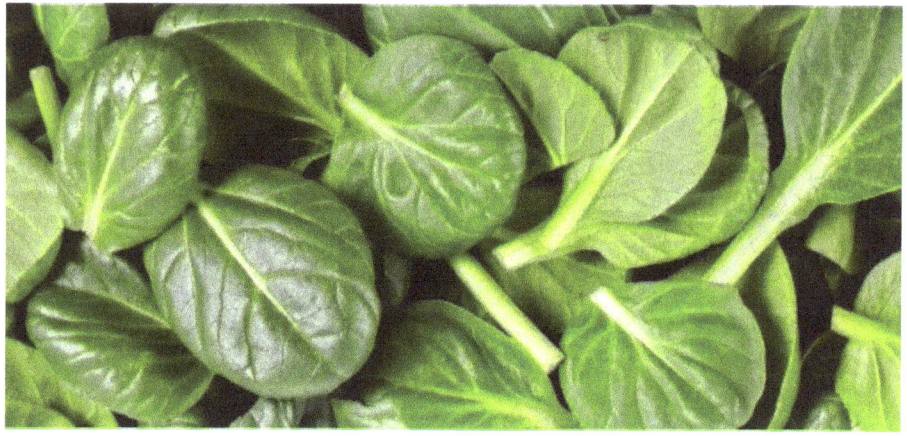

phosphorus for the integrity of bones; dietary fibers that help digestion; muscle-building proteins. Researchers have identified at least 13 different flavonoid compounds in spinach that perform antioxidant functions in the body. Spinach offers a range of physiological benefits, including reduction of inflammation and oxidative stress, promotion of cardiovascular health, and potential mitigation of cancer risk. It serves as an excellent source of essential minerals such as calcium, potassium, magnesium, sulfur, and iron. Due to its considerable protein, carbohydrate, vitamin, and mineral content, incorporating spinach regularly into the diet—particularly in raw forms like smoothies or salads—is recommended. Spinach possesses a comprehensive vitamin profile that supports immune system function and exhibits notable anti-inflammatory effects. Furthermore, its antioxidant compounds facilitate the body's detoxification pathways. The calcium content promotes bone integrity, while iron and magnesium contribute to optimal musculoskeletal performance and may assist in mitigating related nutrient deficiency. Cauliflower, a member of the cruciferous vegetable family like broccoli, shares many beneficial properties with its green counterpart. This widely recognized vegetable deserves a regular place in the diet due to its significant nutritional value, offering essential vitamins, minerals, and antioxidants. Notably, cauliflower is extremely versatile: it can be consumed raw in salads or prepared in a variety of ways, including casseroles, soups, meatloaf, or combined with mashed potatoes. Beyond its culinary appeal, incorporating cauliflower into meals is an effective way to increase nutrient intake. A single serving of cauliflower provides approximately three-quarters of the recommended daily value of vitamin C. Additionally, it supplies vitamin K, proteins, and an array of minerals such as thiamine, riboflavin, niacin, magnesium, phosphorus, vitamin B6, folic acid, pantothenic acid, potassium, and manganese. Cauliflower is rich in vitamins and minerals—including vitamin C, vitamin K, folic acid, and potassium—which contribute to overall health and wellness. It is high in dietary fiber, supporting digestive health, regular bowel function, and the maintenance of healthy intestinal flora. Furthermore, cauliflower contains antioxidants such as glucose plates and isothiocyanate, which help protect the body against free radicals and reduce inflammation.

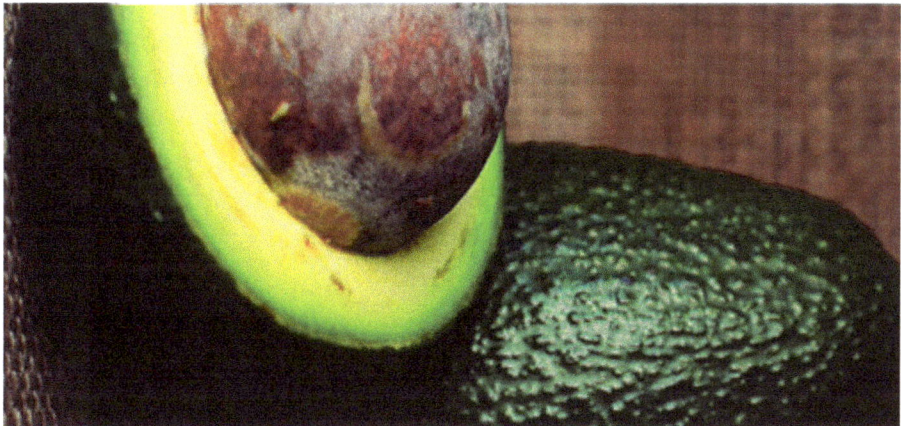

Avocado is a versatile plant classified as both a fruit and a vegetable, with notable applications in nutrition and medicine. It has been associated with beneficial effects on cardiovascular health and serves as an excellent antioxidant due to its rich vitamin content, including vitamins B, C, E, and A. The ripe fruit also provides minerals such as potassium, phosphorus, iron, sodium, calcium, and magnesium. Avocado consumption may assist in the management of eczema and reduction of cholesterol levels. Additionally, avocado oil is valued for nourishing dry or aging skin, attributed primarily to its high concentrations of vitamins A and E. Avocados are most frequently consumed raw, commonly served on toast with garlic and salt, or incorporated into salads.

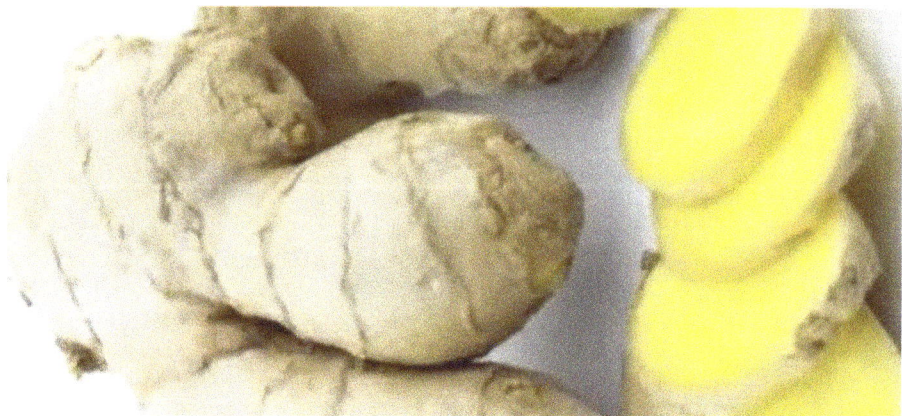

Ginger is a widely utilized natural herb with recognized medicinal properties. Numerous health studies have demonstrated ginger's therapeutic efficacy in addressing various ailments. Characterized by its bitter and pungent flavor profile, ginger is esteemed as a medicinal plant. Its effects remain potent whether consumed fresh, grated, or dried. Documented benefits include antispasmodic, anti-nausea, anti-fungal, anti-inflammatory, antiseptic, antibacterial, antiviral, and antitussive qualities. Ginger is also a significant source of vitamins A, C, E, and B complex, in addition to containing substantial amounts of magnesium, phosphorus, potassium, sodium, iron, zinc, calcium, and beta-carotene. The root can be consumed fresh or dried, making it a valuable option for those seeking natural remedies. Among its many benefits, ginger is particularly noted for its role in supporting immune system function.

Cavolo Nero vegetable is a member of the cabbage family and serves as an excellent source of essential vitamins during winter, particularly due to its superior cold tolerance compared to conventional cabbage. Originating from Asia and historically referred to as Italian cabbage in early documents, it provides significant nutritional value. A single serving supplies the recommended daily intake of vitamins A and C, while also offering vitamins

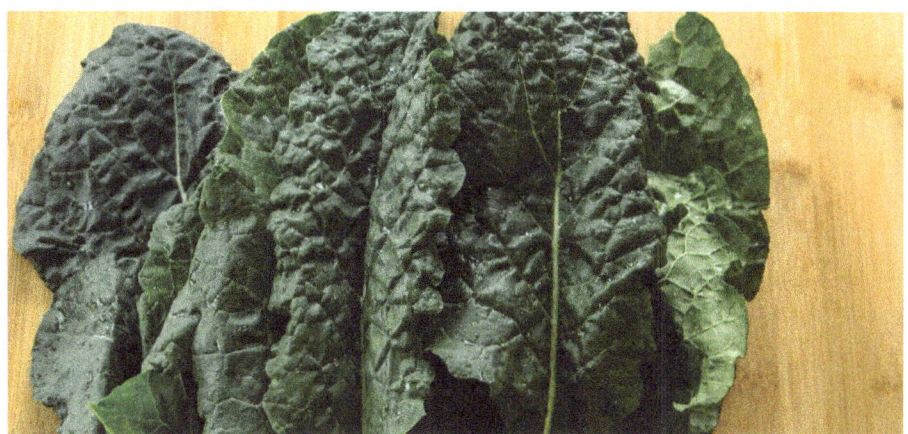

B1, B2, E, as well as notable amounts of protein, carbohydrates, and dietary fiber that aid digestion. It contains substantial quantities of vital mineral salts, including calcium, potassium, magnesium, sulfur, and iron. The antioxidant content supports the body's detoxification processes, and its calcium contributes to bone health. Due to its high nutrient density and low caloric content, it is suitable for those following a calorie-controlled diet. Consuming it raw is recommended to preserve its nutritional properties.

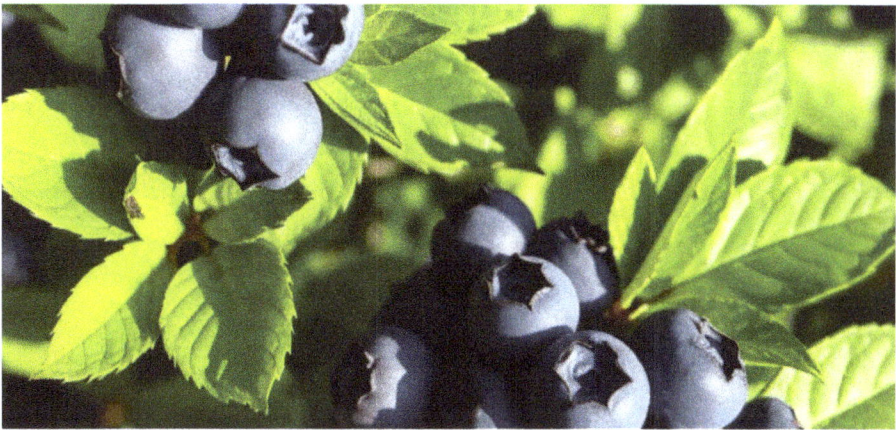

Blueberries are recognized for possessing some of the highest antioxidant levels among commonly consumed fruits and vegetables. Their popularity is largely attributed to their culinary versatility, serving as a frequent ingredient in various desserts featuring forest fruits, such as cakes and ice creams. Native to Northern Europe, blueberries thrive at elevations reaching 2,500 meters. The presence of minerals such as iron, phosphorus, calcium, manganese, zinc, and vitamin K in blueberries plays an integral role in supporting bone health and strength. Iron and zinc are essential for maintaining bone and joint integrity. Inadequate vitamin K intake is associated with increased risk of fractures, whereas sufficient consumption enhances calcium processing and reduces vitamin K depletion. Additionally, the fiber, potassium, folic acid, vitamin C, vitamin B6, and phytonutrients in blueberries collectively contribute to cardiovascular health; for instance, fiber contributes to lower blood cholesterol levels, thereby reducing the risk of heart disease. Vitamins C and A found in blueberries serve to protect cells, inhibit tumor development, reduce systemic inflammation, and slow the progression of various cancers, including lung, oral, pharyngeal, uterine, and prostate cancers. Folic acid is also involved in DNA synthesis and repair, mitigating the emergence of cancer cells associated with DNA mutations. Regular blueberry consumption has been shown to slow cognitive decline and may reduce the risk of developing Parkinson's disease.

Favorite recipes

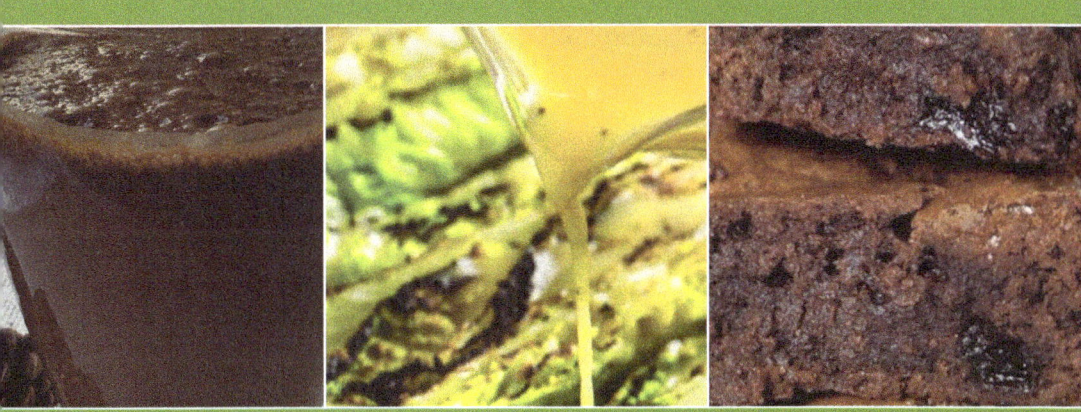

Food intolerance and how to deal with it

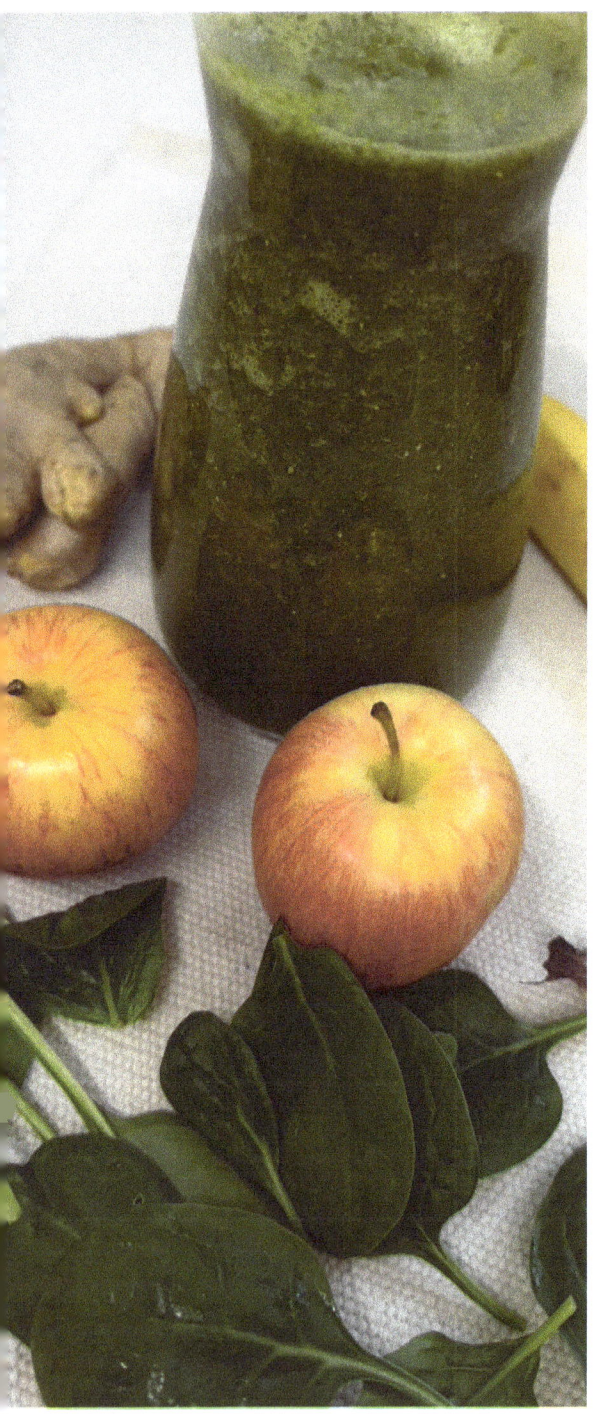

Green smoothie

Ingredients:
260g spinach
1 banana
2 apples
2 slices of ginger
2 slices of lemon
Pinch of matcha

Method: add spinach/ apples/ banana /ginger and lemon to the blender. Fill it up with water until covers them all. Blend it for 2-4 minutes.

Citrus juice

Ingredients:
3 slices of pineapple
2 apples
1 lemon
3 slices of ginger (even more)
1 bunch of mint leaves

Methods: add all items in the juicer. Serve it with ice.

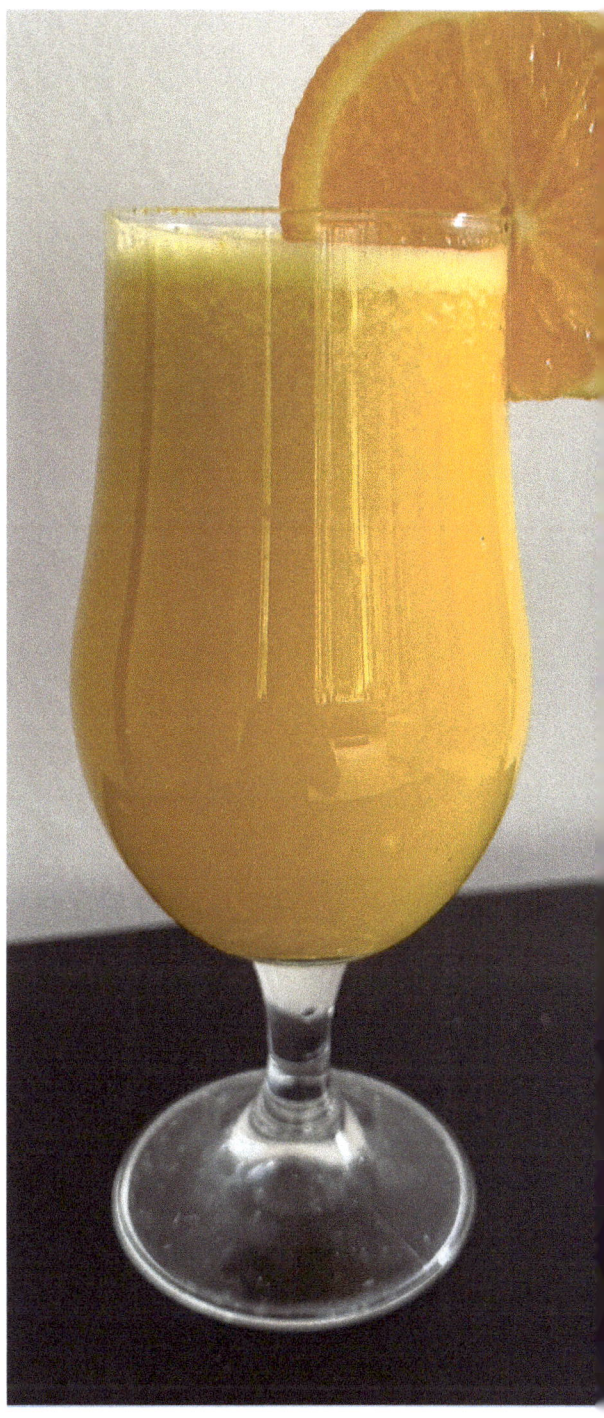

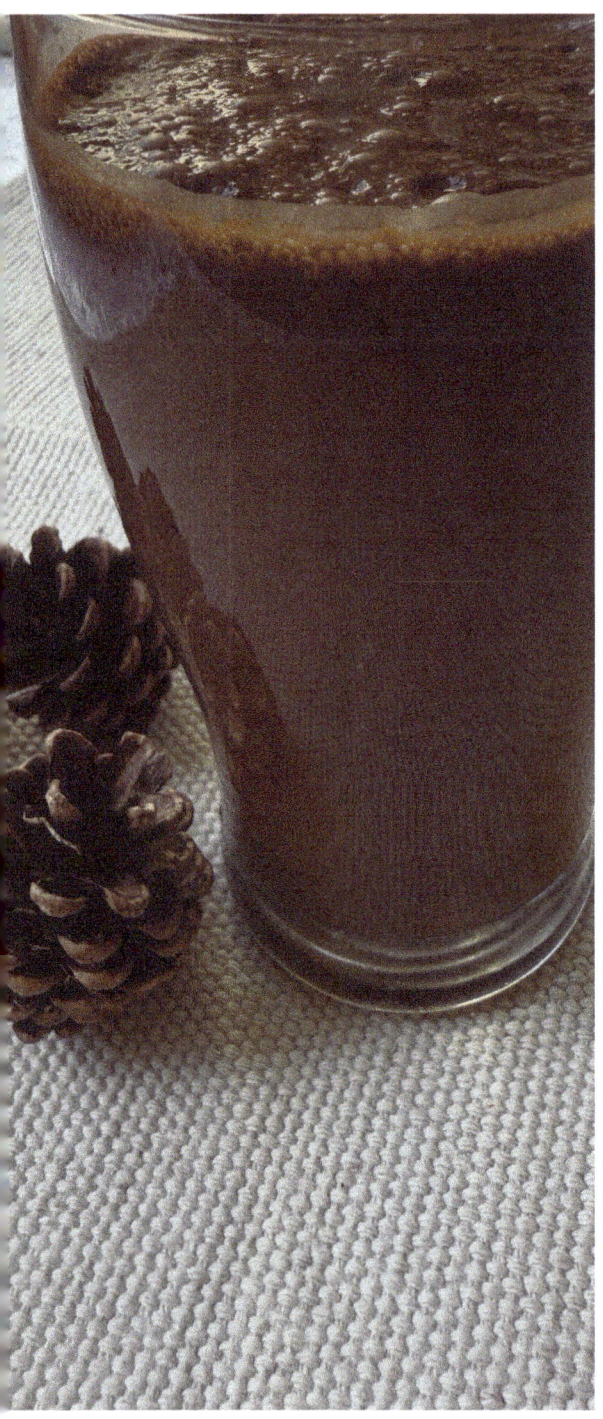

Chocolate smoothie

Ingredients:
2 teaspoons of cacao powder
1 teaspoon of chia seeds
2 bananas
half cup of blueberry
coconut milk

Methods: add all ingredients in a blender.

Top up with coconut milk and blend it for 2-3 minutes.

Fresh juice

Ingredients:
2 bunches of celery sticks
2 slices of fresh ginger
1 lemon

Methods: Juice it with the juicer. Served cold.

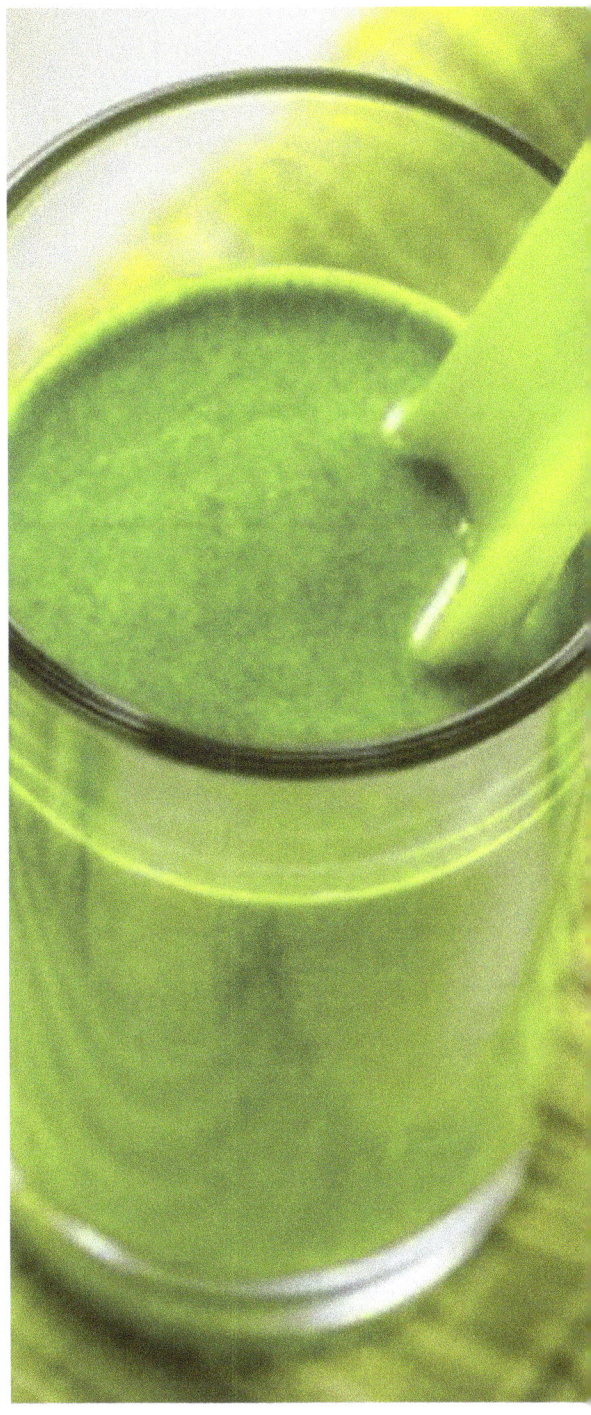

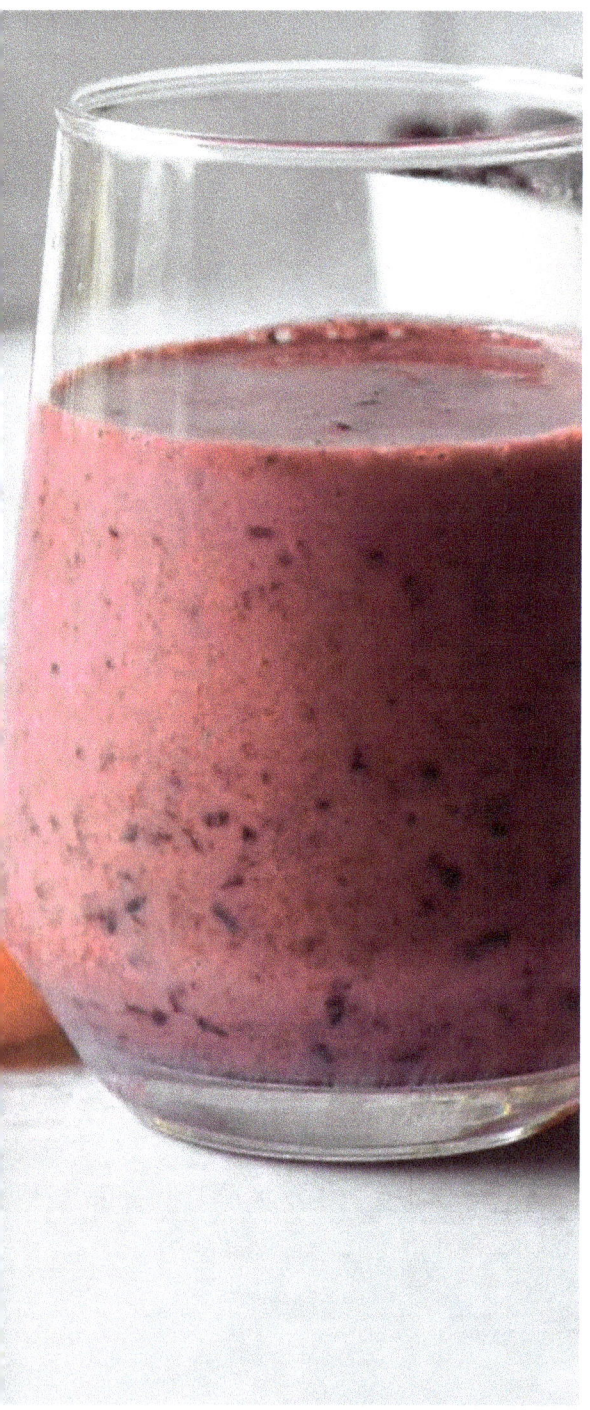

Red Smoothie

Ingredients:
1 cup of berry
1 small cauliflower
2 small beetroots
1 banana
1 teaspoon of Goji berry
coconut water

Methods: add all in a blender, top up with coconut water.

Blend it for 2-3 minutes.

Rainbow salat dressing

Ingredients:
3 dates
1 squeezed lemon
1 raw medium tomato
Pinch of chilly or chilly cream
½ teaspoon of honey
10g dill
1 teaspoon nutritional yeast
½ teaspoon coconut liquid amino acid
Few drops of pomegranate molasses
Pinch of salt and pepper

Methods: add all ingredients in blender and mix them for 2-3 minutes. Add on top of the salad this mixture. Pumpkin seeds are on choice.

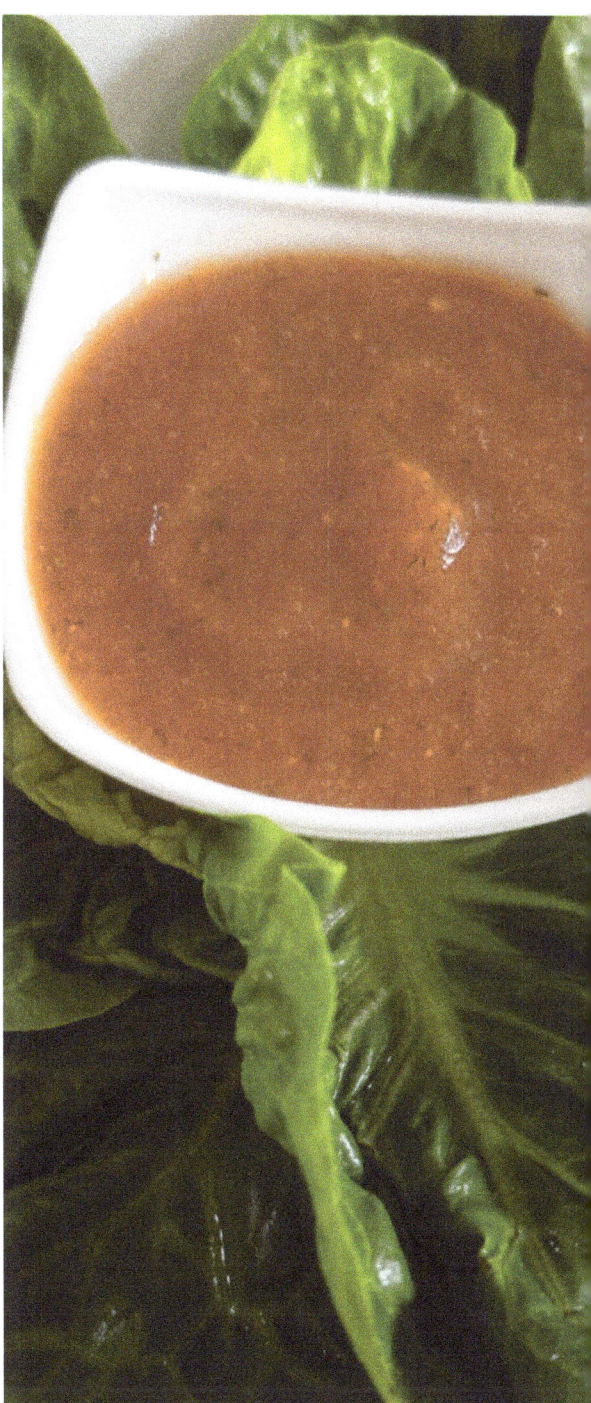

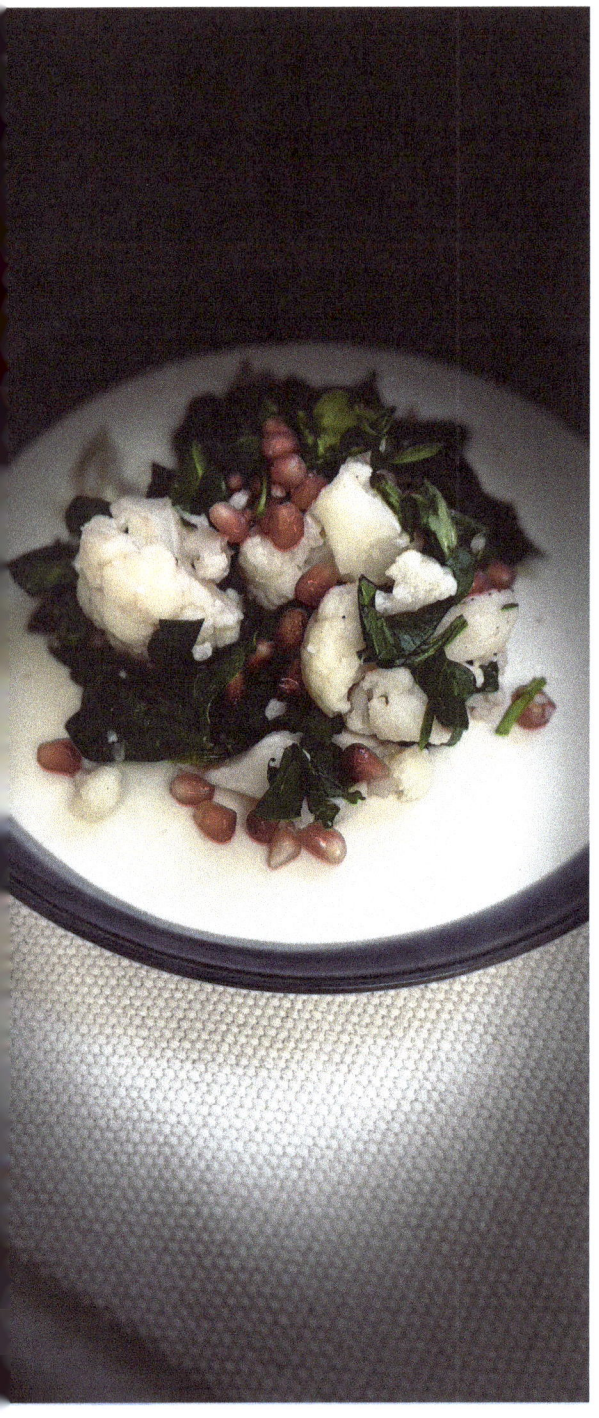

Mix and match

Ingredients:
1 head of cauliflower
1 pomegranate
1 handful of spinach
Pinch of salt
Pinch of mixed pepper
5 drops of coconut aminos organic (lemon as substitute)

Methods: boil the cauliflower in water. Place it in a bowl where you add the spinach, salt, pepper, coconut aminos and pomegranate. (the pomegranate needs to be broke open and take the seeds out, only use the seeds). Mixed them up.

Favorite recipes

Pineapple with coconut and mint drizzle salad

Ingredients:
1 medium ripe pineapple, skin removed
1 teaspoon honey
100mg coconut yoghurt
Pinch of sea salt/ pinch of pepper
Squeeze 1 lemon/or lime
Mint leaves (25mg pack)
Chilly powder or chilly sauce

Methods: cut pineapple in small pieces, place them in a bowl. Cut up the mint in small and tuck it between the pineapples. Add coconut yoghurt, salt, pepper, chilly, lemon, honey in a blender. Mix it for 2 minutes. Add on top of the pineapple. Serve it chilled.

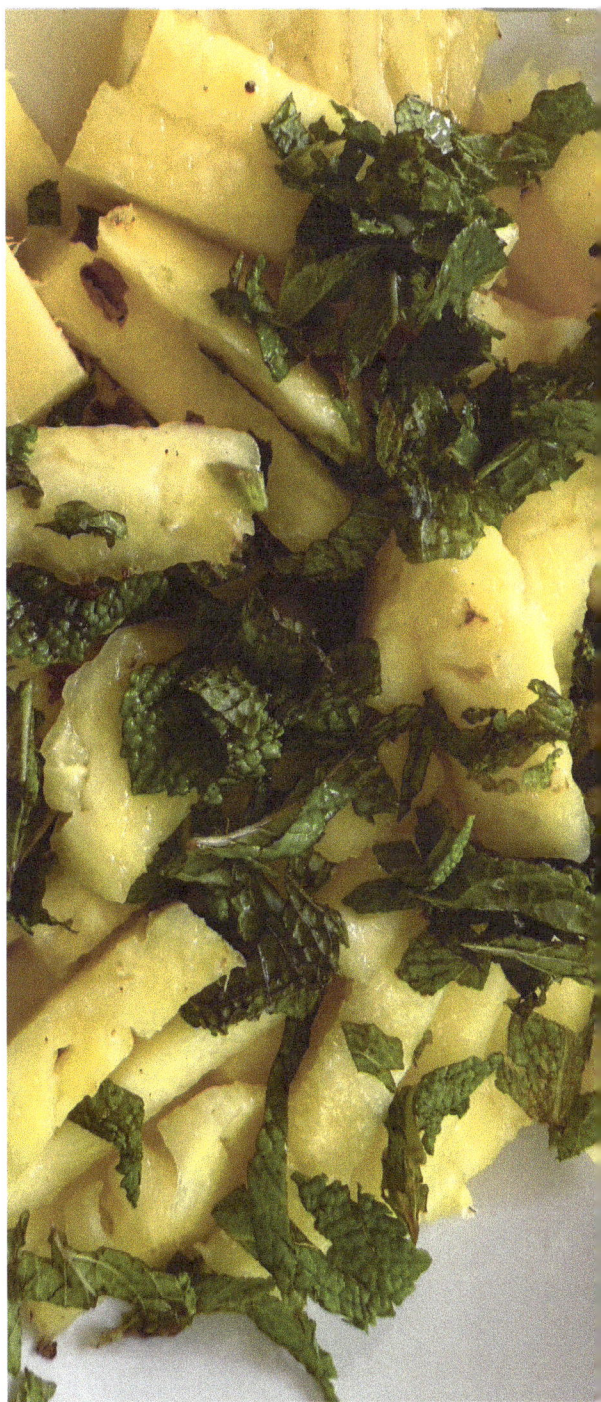

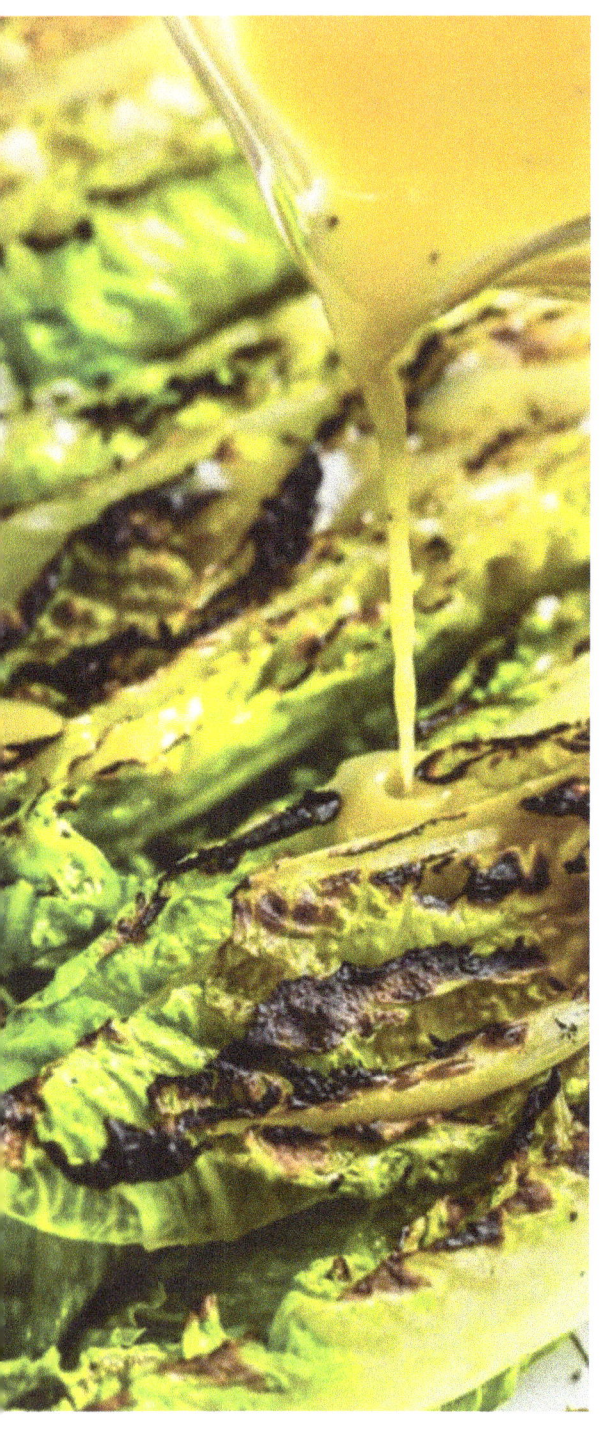

Hot salad

Ingredients:
2 little gem lettuces
2 cloves garlic
1 shallot onion
vegetable stock (250mg)
few sprigs thyme
1 lemon (juiced)
Gluten free bread croutons

Dressing:
1 teaspoon mustard
chili powder or chili sauce
1 teaspoon of coconut aminos acid organic
20g pack tarragon leaves finely chopped
2 tablespoon coconut yoghurt
salt and pepper

Methods: add the washed lettuces, cut side down, in a hot pan add garlic and fry over a medium high heat until golden (4-6 minutes), then pour in the vegetable stock, thyme, lemon and chilly and simmer for few minutes. Add to a blender and pour it over the salads. Add croutons.

Favorite recipes

Fermented (pickled) mixed vegetable

Ingredients:
1 small cauliflower
1 small red cabbage
2 big tablespoons of sea salt
2 ½ liter of water
1 teaspoon grain black pepper
1 small white onion
2 small carrots
1 small bunch dill
10 mg thymes
3 thick slices of root horseradish

Methods: cut cauliflower in small pieces, then shred the red cabbage, cut up in slices the onion and carrots add all in a jug (3kg) add between the layer's add dill and thyme, top up the jug with them. Boil 2 ½ kg of water for 10 min, add the pepper salt. Let it cool. Top up the jug full of vegetables with the water. To be served in 5-7 days.

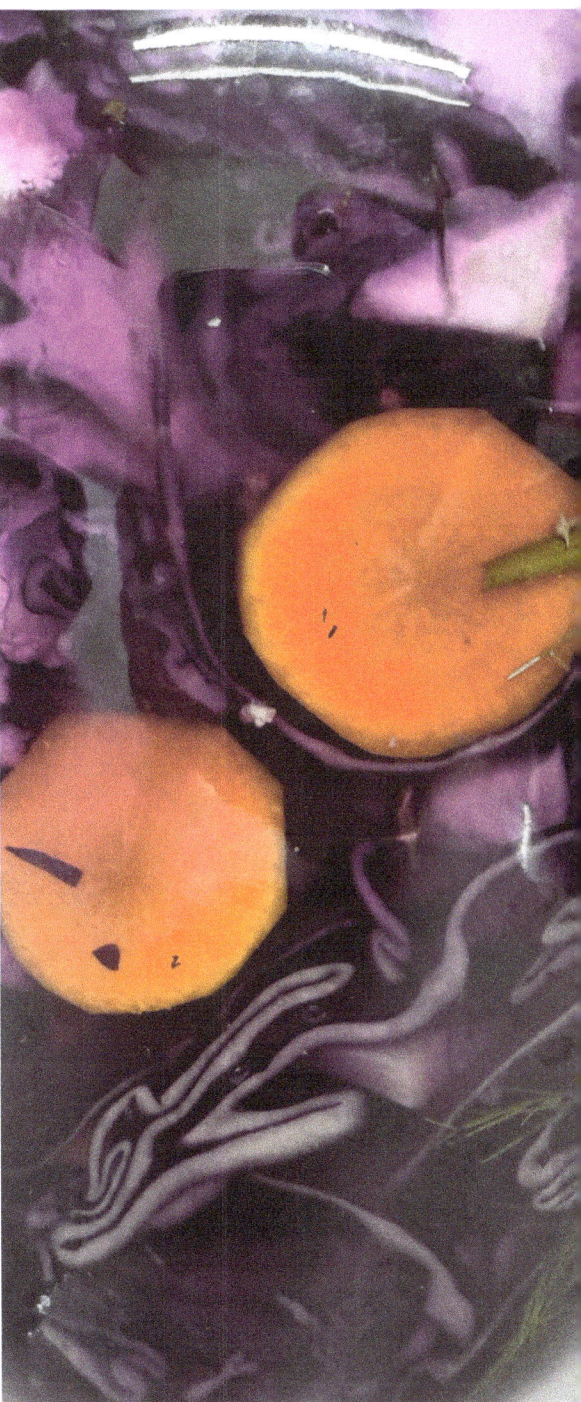

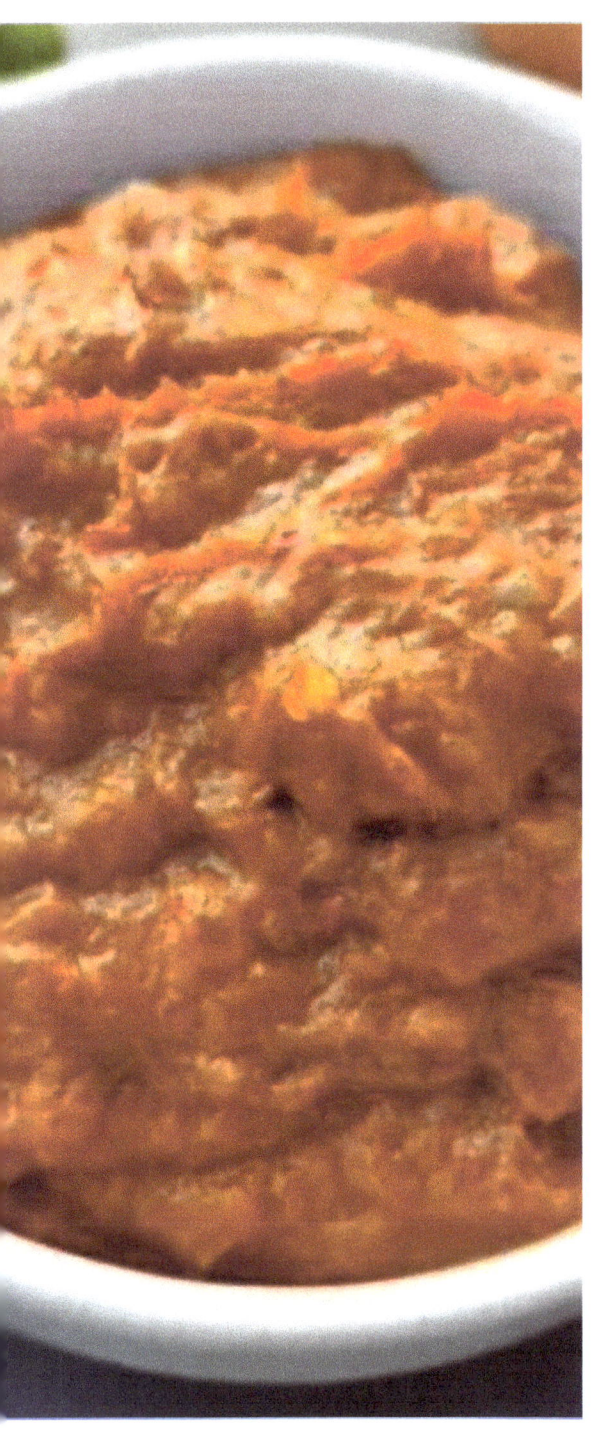

Roasted vegetable spread

Ingredients:
3 red peppers
1 eggplant
1 onion
½ l water
pinch of salt
punch of grain black pepper
2/3 bay leafs

Methods: cut all vegetables in small pieces. Add them in a pan and roast them for 10 minutes in the oven. Take a medium saucepan, add all vegetables and the water, pepper, salt, 2-3 bay leaf's and simmer it for the next 20 minutes. Remove bay leafs and blend it. Serve it warm or cold on toast.

Chia taramasalata

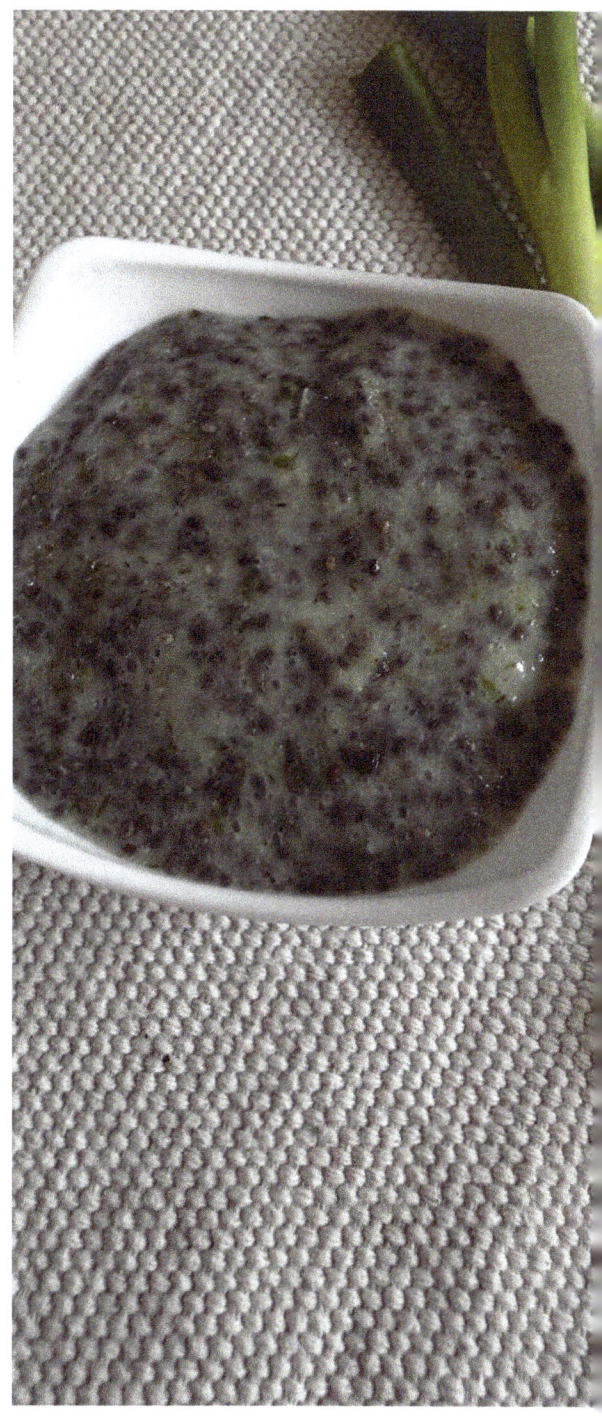

Ingredients:
half cup of chia seeds
1 small cup of coconut milk
10g chives
pinch of salt and pepper
½ teaspoon nutritional yeast

Methods: leave chia seeds in coconut milk overnight, then add all ingredients in a mixer, mixed them for 2 minutes and enjoy it on a toast with garlic.

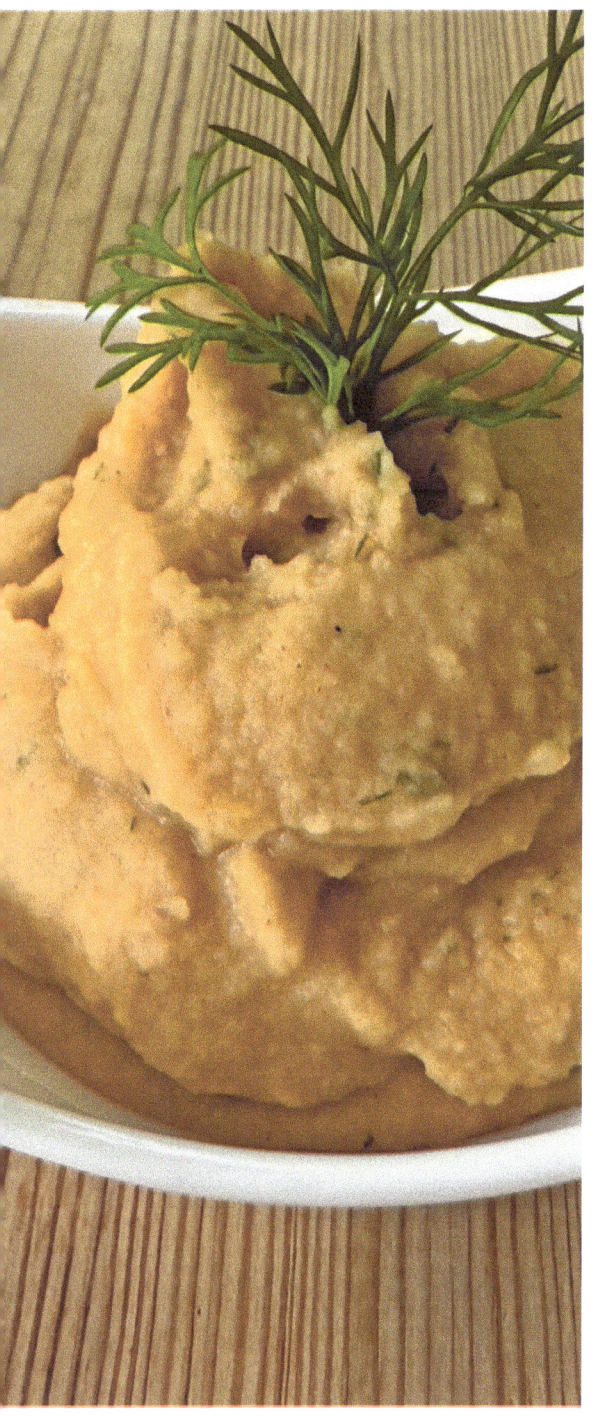

Lentils pate

Ingredients
500mg red lentil
1 pinch of tandoori masala
pinch of salt and pepper
2/3 scallion stalk
3 teaspoons of red wine
1/2 lemon
4 large spoons of water

Methods: cook the red lentils until soft, then add all the above ingredients and spices, then mix until creamy.

Eggplant spread

Ingredients:
2 eggplants
½ teaspoon mustard
pinch of salt and pepper
1 pinch chilly
½ teaspoon nutritional yeast
10g chives

Methods: add eggplant to oven for 30 minutes. Peel it off and put it with all the other ingredients to a blender and mix it up. Spread it on toast or bagels.

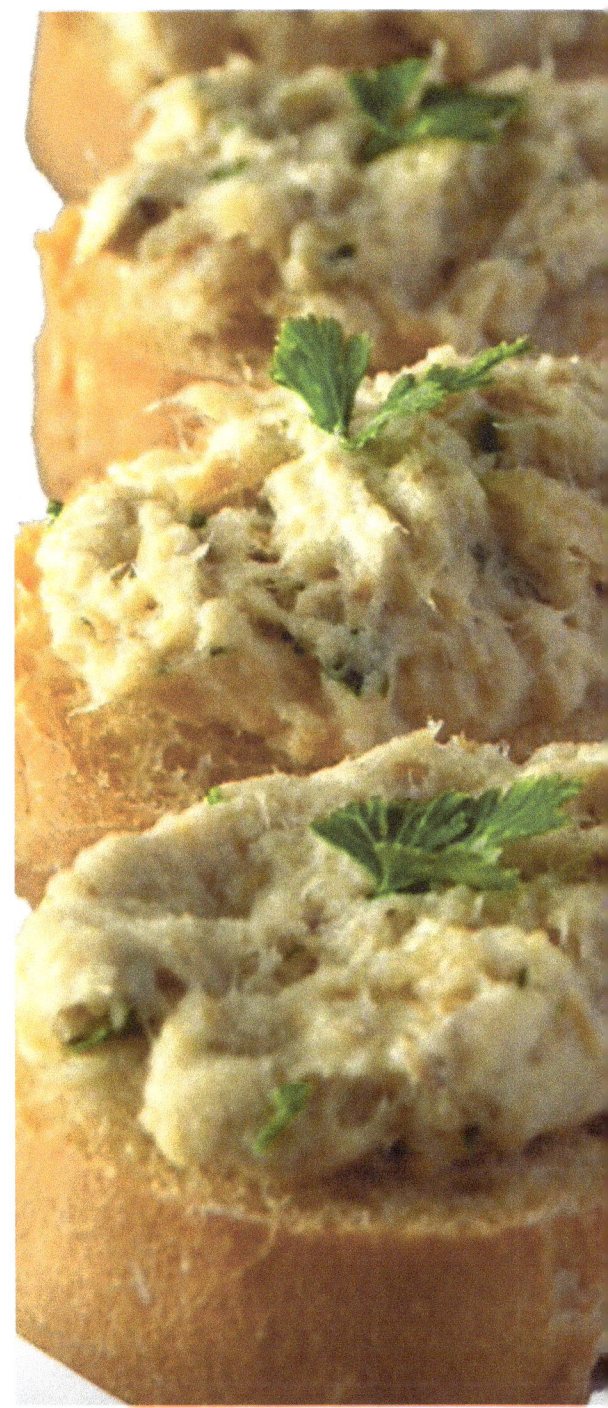

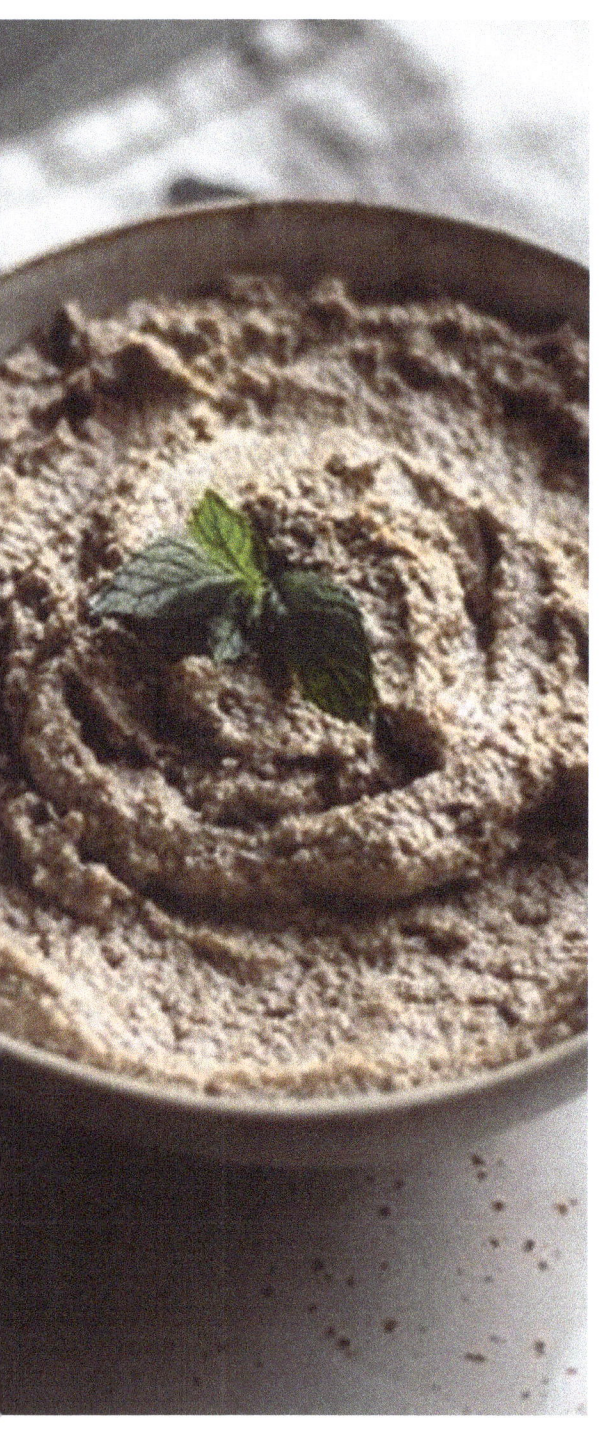

Roasted mushroom spread

Ingredients:
6 medium mushrooms (any)
1 medium onion
1 tablespoon of rice (any)
1 tablespoon avocado
1/2 clove garlic
2 thyme threads
4 tablespoons of water
pinch of salt and pepper

Methods: add mushrooms and onion with garlic in the oven, bake it for 15-20 minutes on low heat. Boil the rice for 15 minutes. When done add all in a blender and mix them together. Mix it until it's a smooth paste. Serve it cold or warm.

Celery soup

Ingredients:
1 small celeriac
1 medium white onion
3 big potatoes
1 medium apple
½ bay leafs
½ pieces of tarragon in the end
pinch of salt
pinch of black pepper
water (2l)

Methods: cut all vegetables in small pieces, washed them well and add them into the boiling water, add salt and pepper add bay leafs. Boil it for 20 minutes than add tarragon. When cooled, remove bay leafs, then mixed them up in a blender for 2 minutes.

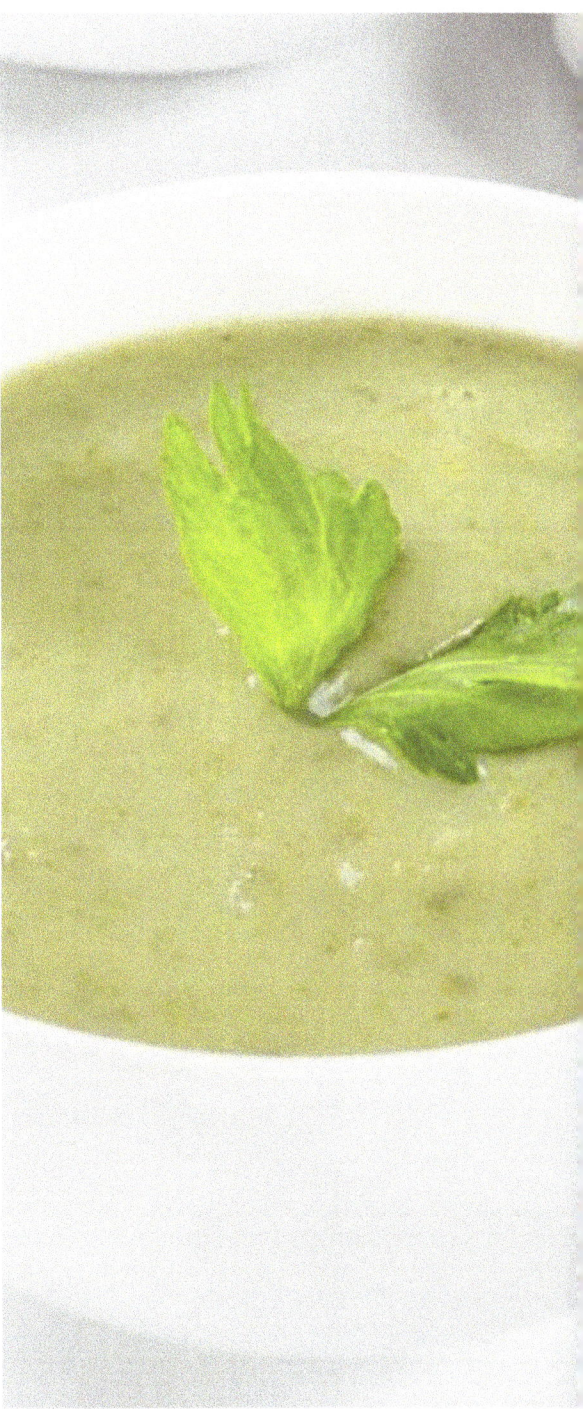

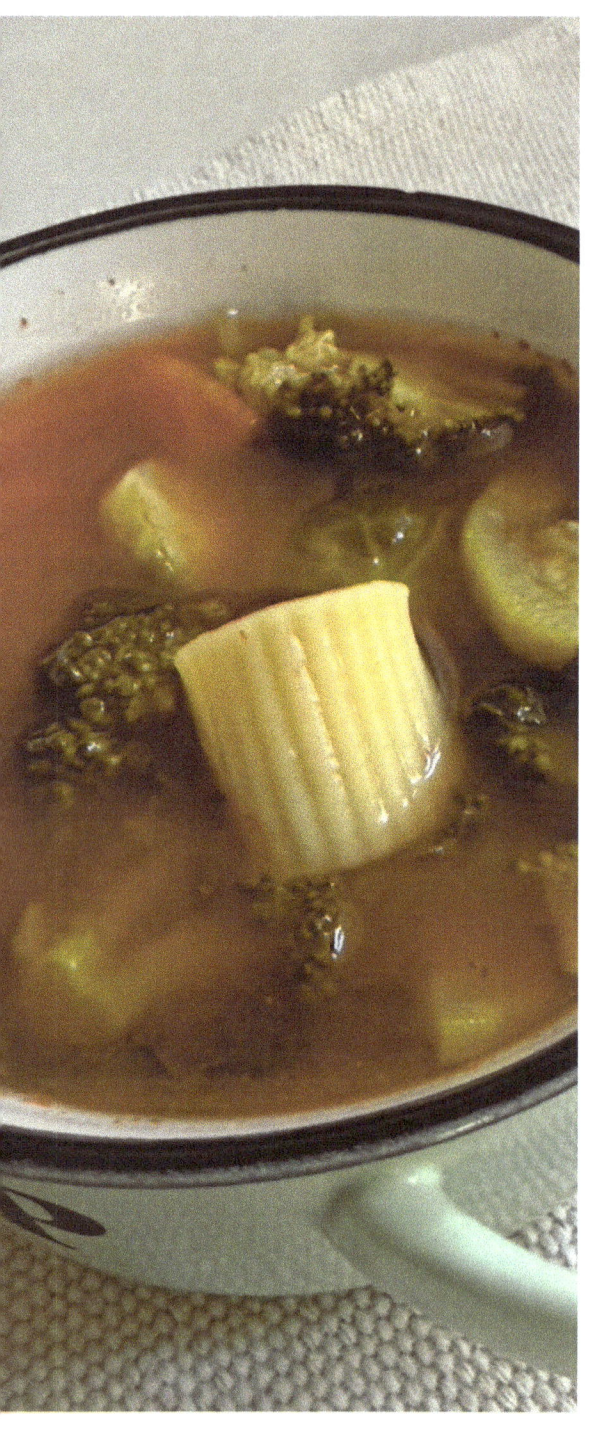

"My minestrone" soup

Ingredients:
2 small carrots
1 celery stick
1 small white onion
1 small courgette
1 leaf of kale
pinch of oregano
pinch of salt
pinch of black pepper
Gluten free pasta (handful)
Organic tomato paste (half of a cup)
2 bay leafs
Water (2l)

Methods: Wash and cut all vegetables in small pieces. Add them in boiling water, add the pasta and bay leafs with seasoning. Boil the soup for 25 minutes. Add the organic tomato paste in the end and boil it for the next 3-4 minutes

Favorite recipes

Parsnip soup

Ingredients:
1 small parsnip
1 small apple
3 small potatoes
1 small shallot
1 celery stick
pinch of salt
pinch of black pepper
2 tablespoons of nutritional yeast
Parsley leaves (10mg from pack)
1 tablespoon coconut amino acid liquid
water

Methods: cut small pieces all vegetables, add salt, pepper, nutritional yeast, parsley, aminos coconut and boil them for 20 minutes. Mixed all in a blender for 2 minutes. Add chili flakes on top when served.

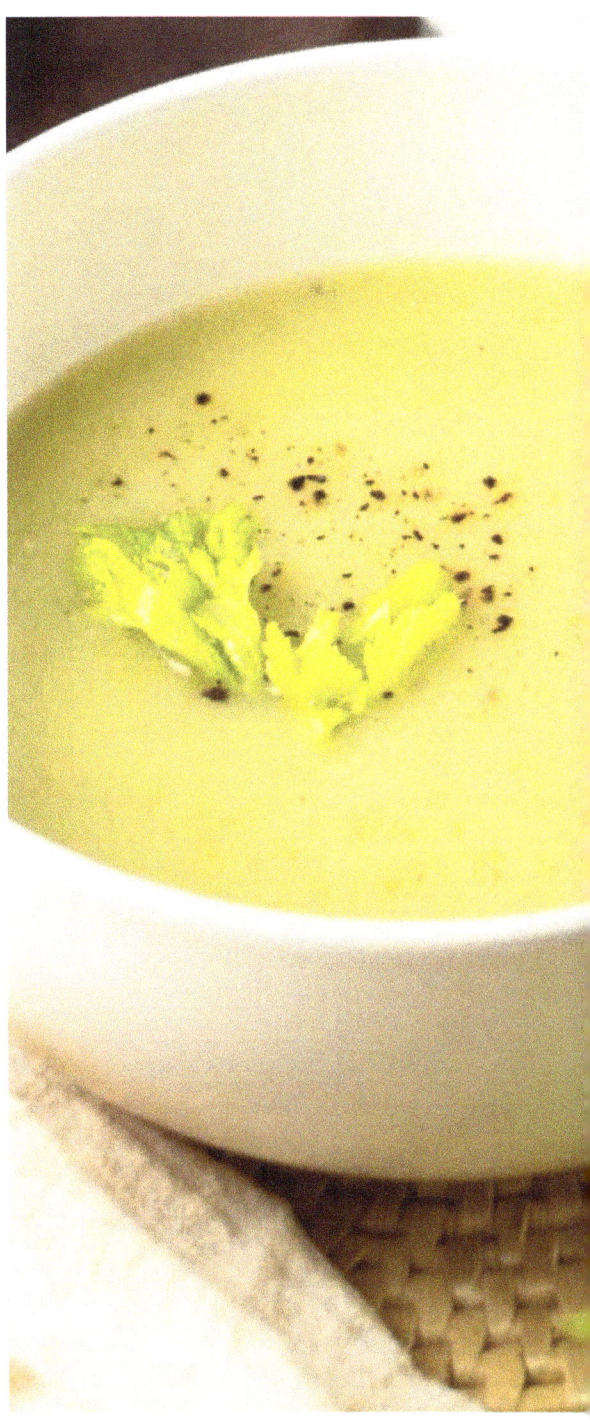

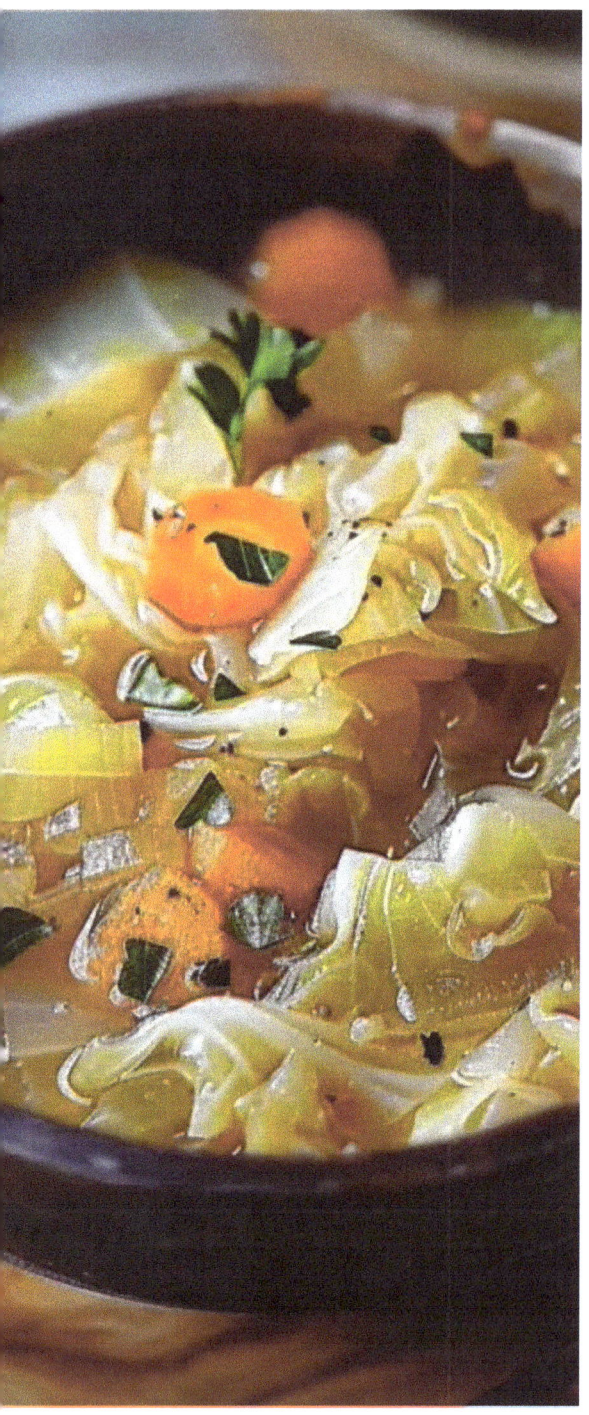

Sour soup

Ingredients:
1 small red onion
2 small carrots
fermented cabbage (500mg)
lovage (10mg from pack)
sweet paprika one pinch
Sauerkraut juice ½ cup
water (2l)

Methods: wash and cut in small pieces the carrots and the onion, add in boiling water for 15 minutes than add the cabbage and boil it for the next 15 minutes. Add lovage, sweet paprika, salt and pepper and sauerkraut juice in the end.

Favorite recipes

Roasted red pepper cream soup

Ingredients:
4-5 red peppers
1 red onion
1 clove garlic
2 medium potatoes
10g rosemary
10g thyme
1 pinch salt and pepper on choice
water

Methods: add peppers, garlic, onion, sprinkle the rosemary and thyme over the pepper and onion, put them in the oven for the next 15 min. Boil potatoes for 10 minutes, add salt and pepper. Put them together in a bowl and boil them all in the water for further 15 minutes. Blend them all together to become a crème soup. Serve it with gluten free croutons.

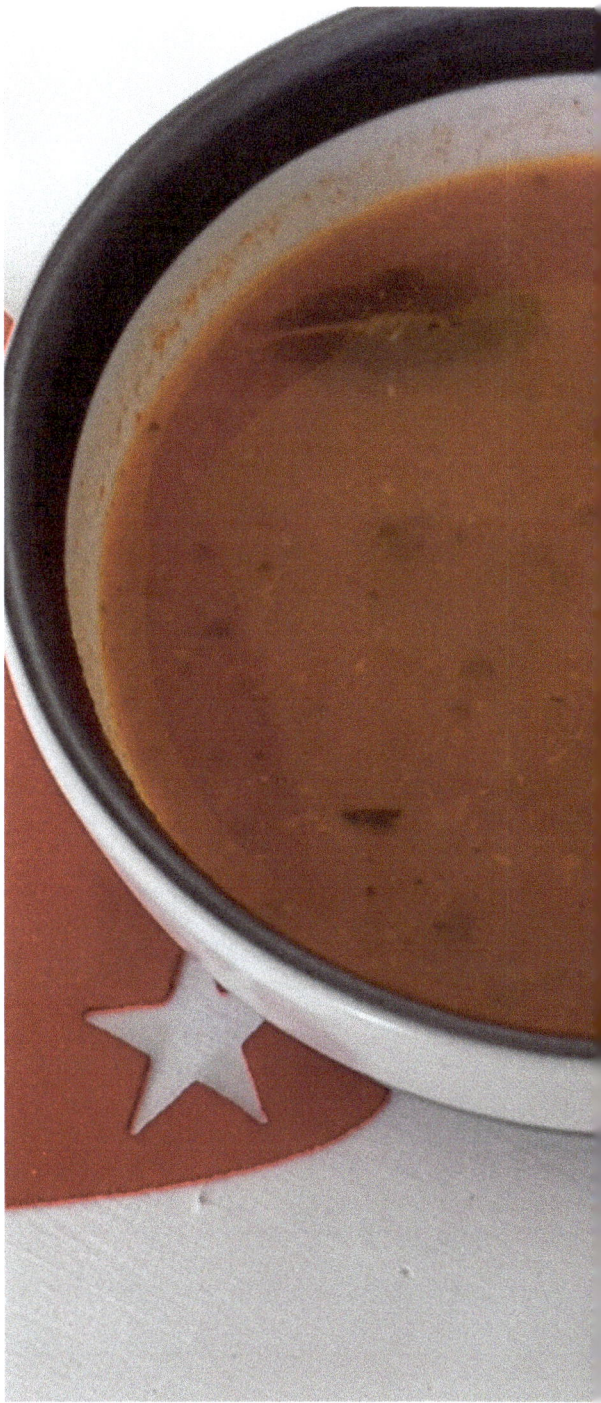

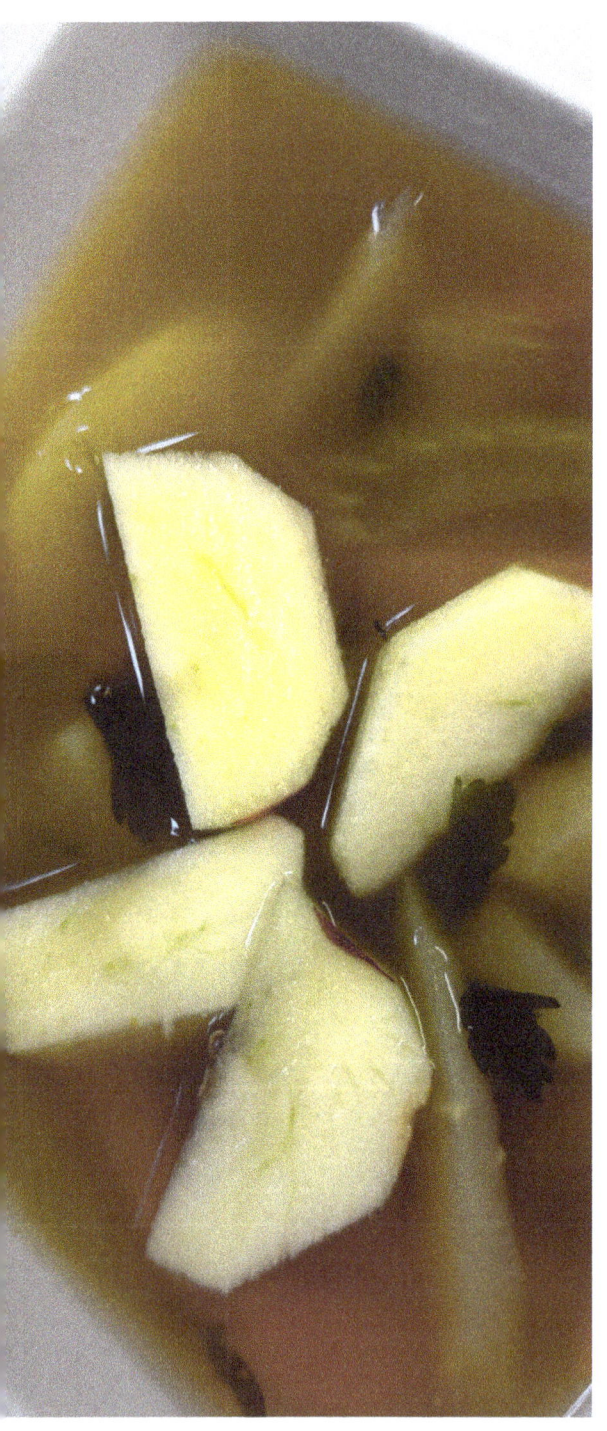

Vegetable soup with apple

Ingredients:
1 medium onion
2 medium potatoes
small broccoli
1 apple
vermicelli noodles half pack (on choice)
10g parsley leaves
10g lovage
pinch of salt and pepper
water

Methods: add in hot water the onion, potatoes, broccoli, apple (cut them in small pieces all of them) and boil it for 20 minutes.

Add vermicelli noodles, salt and pepper, parsley and lovage and boil them for the next 10 minutes. Serve it hot.

Stuffed kohlrabi

Ingredients:
1 small kohlrabi
1 small shallot
1 clove garlic
1 medium potato
handful of spinach
pinch of salt and pepper

Methods: peel kohlrabi and scrub out the middle of kohlrabi, make a medium hole. Fill in the kohlrabi with grated potato, (chop up) onion, the spinach and garlic, salt and pepper. Put the filled kohlrabi in the casserole dish and put in the oven on 180 Celsius for 25 minutes, then take off the top of the casserole and put it back in the oven for next 10 minutes. Serve it with coconut yoghurt on top

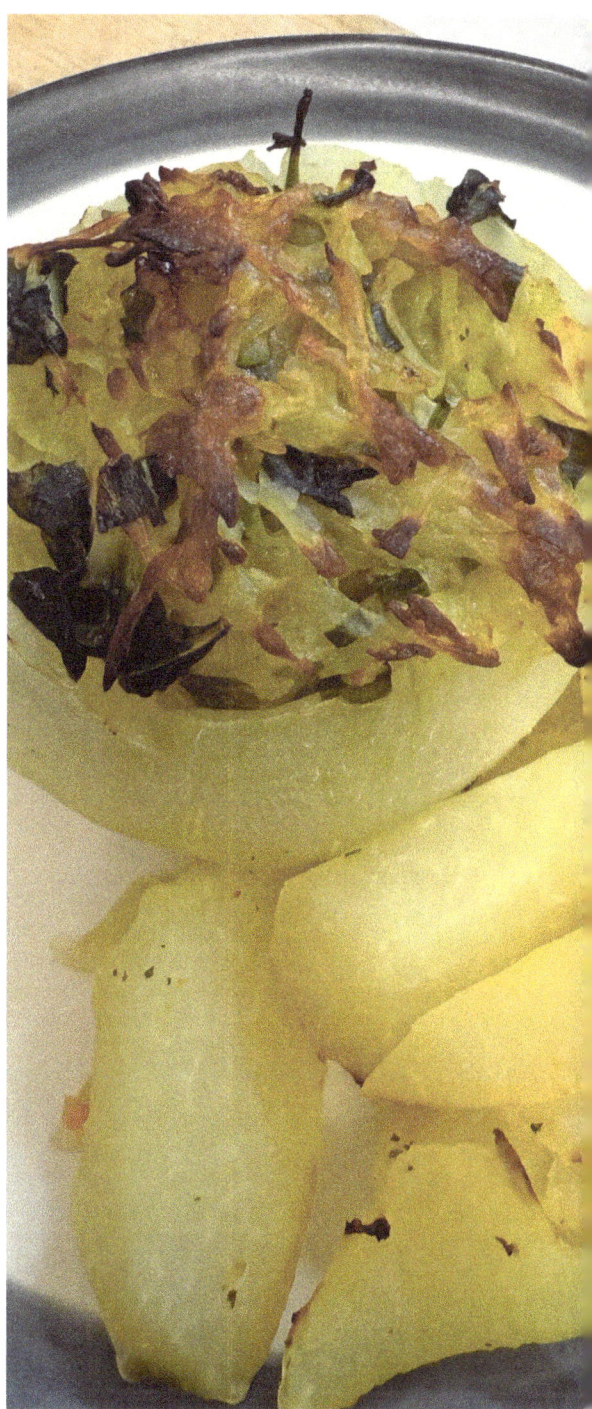

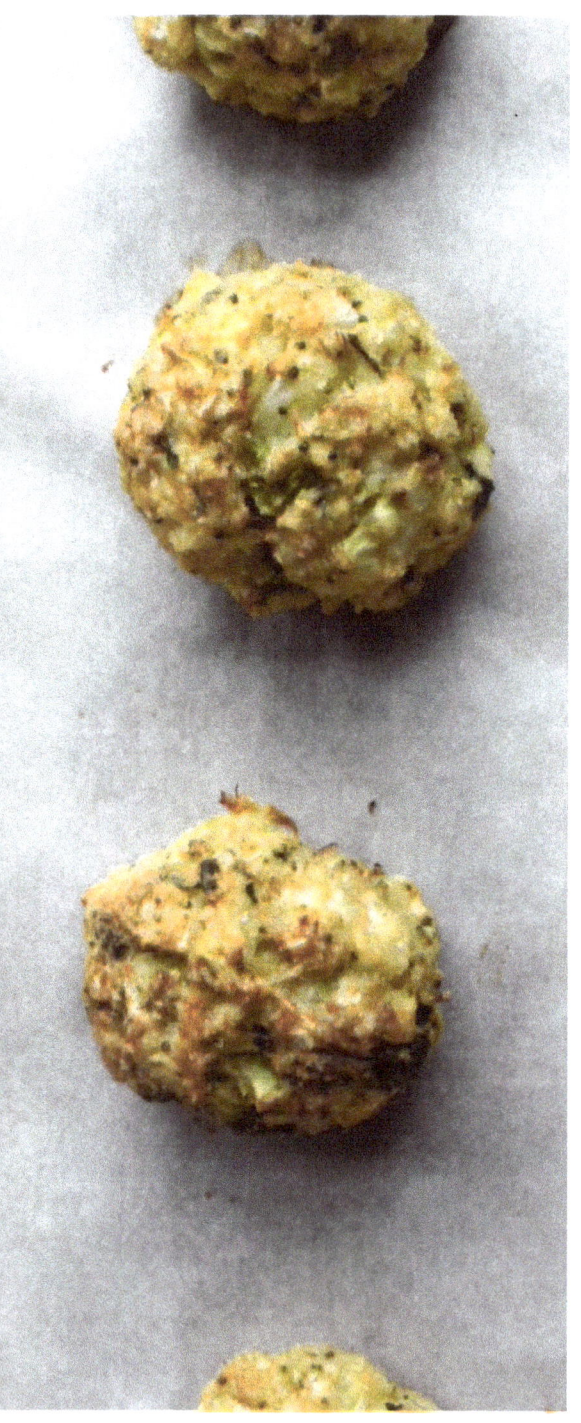

Broccoli balls

Ingredients:
1 medium broccoli
1 bunch chives
½ cup of gluten free breadcrumbs
1 spoon of nutritional yeast
pepper and salt by taste
chilly

Methods: steam broccoli and chopped them in very small pieces along with the chives, add the crumbs, nutritional yeast, salt, pepper, chilly. Mixed them, make small balls, add them in the air fryer for 20 minutes.

Favorite recipes

Cottage pie

Ingredients:
3 medium potatoes
1 carrot
1 medium onion
3 medium mushrooms
100g tomatoes pure
pinch salt and pepper
150g coconut milk
2 bay leafs
thyme 10g
pinch of nutmeg

Methods: add potatoes to boil for 20 minutes, add milk and mash it up. Add all other ingredients in sous pan and leave it to cook for 15 minutes. Add all ingredients from sous pan to a casserole dish, add on top the mash potato with a pinch of nutmeg. Leave it in the oven for 15-20 min.

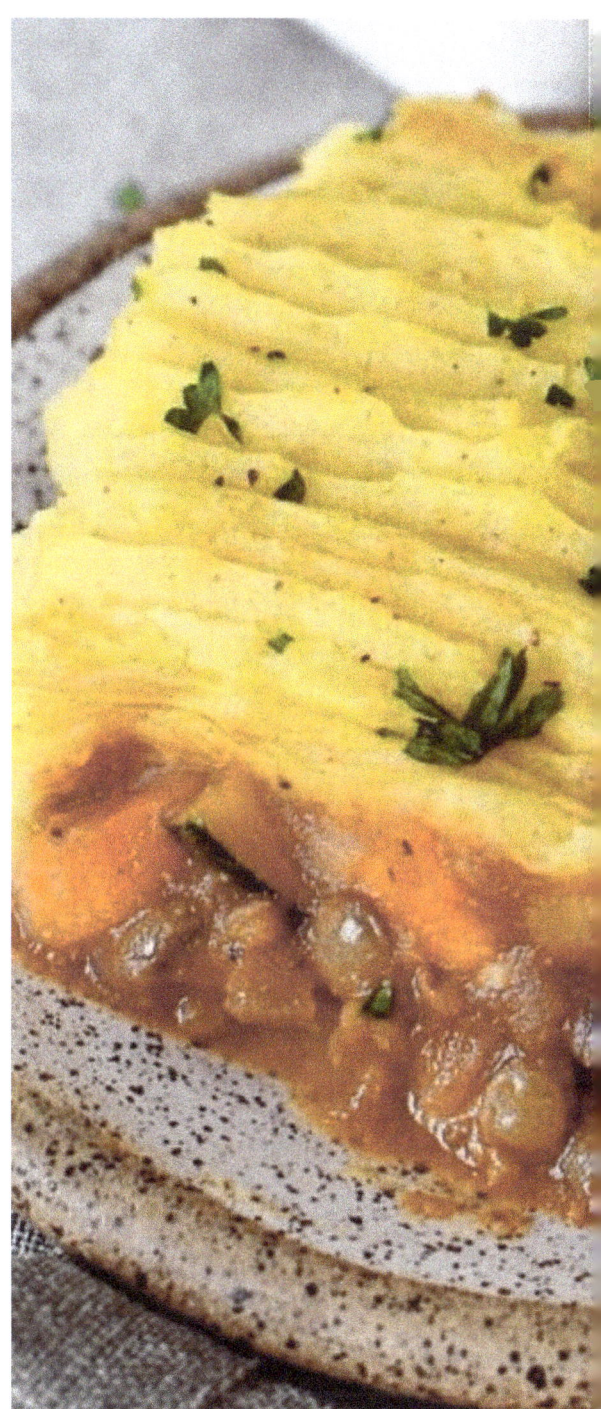

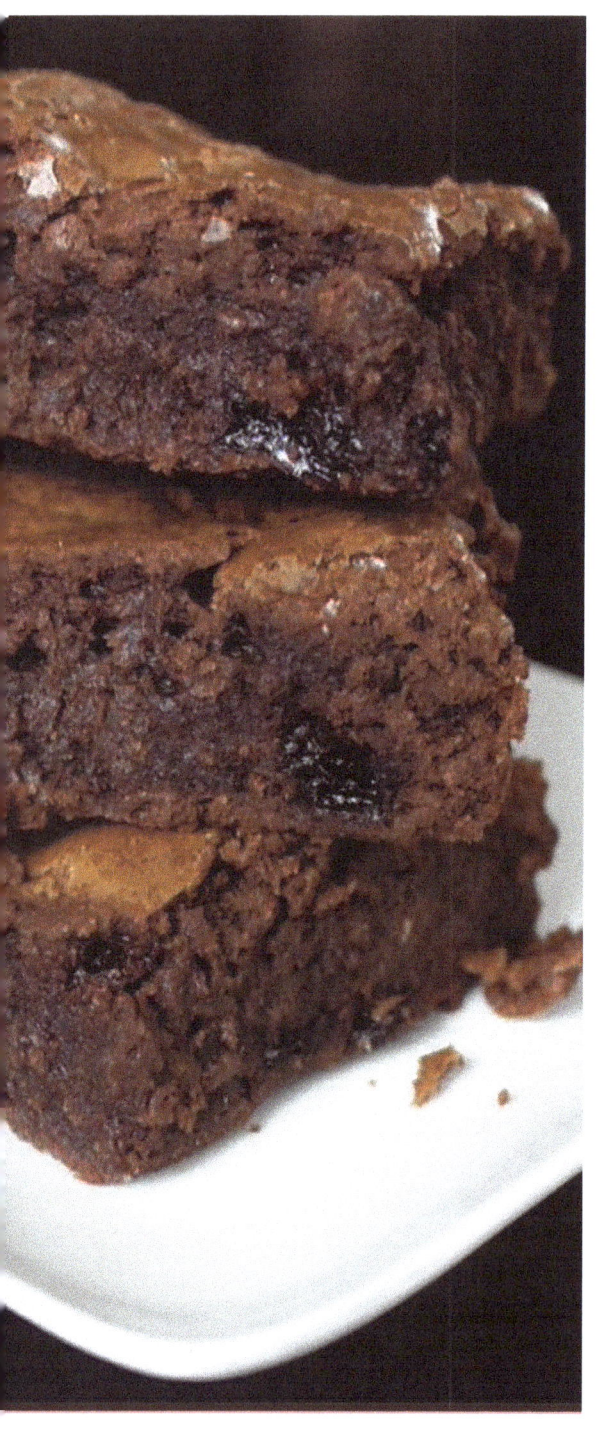

Gluten free brownies

Ingredients:
1 cup gluten free flour
4 small chocolate chips
1 cup coconut milk
1 sachet baking powder
2 tablespoon cocoa powder
1 tablespoon of coconut sugar
1 spoon rum essence
1 teaspoon of raisins
 pinch of table salt
pinch of cinnamon and allspice

Methods: put all the above in a casserole stir it well until it's smooth and leave it in the oven for 35 minutes on 180C. Add coconut ice cream on top.

Mojito nonalcoholic

Ingredients:
10 mint leaves
2 teaspoons of coconut sugar
½ lime
250 ml sparkling water

Methods: crush mint leaves and sugar, add lime, pour sparkling water add ice, serve with a straw, garnish with mint leaves or lemon slices.

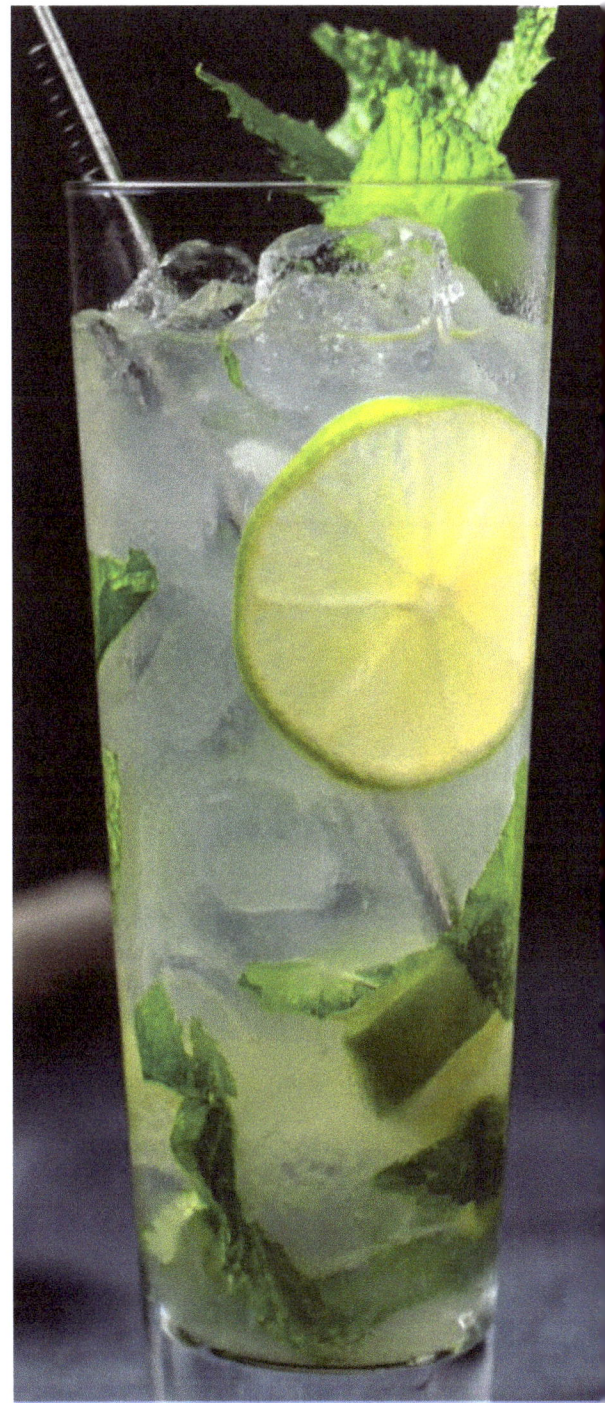

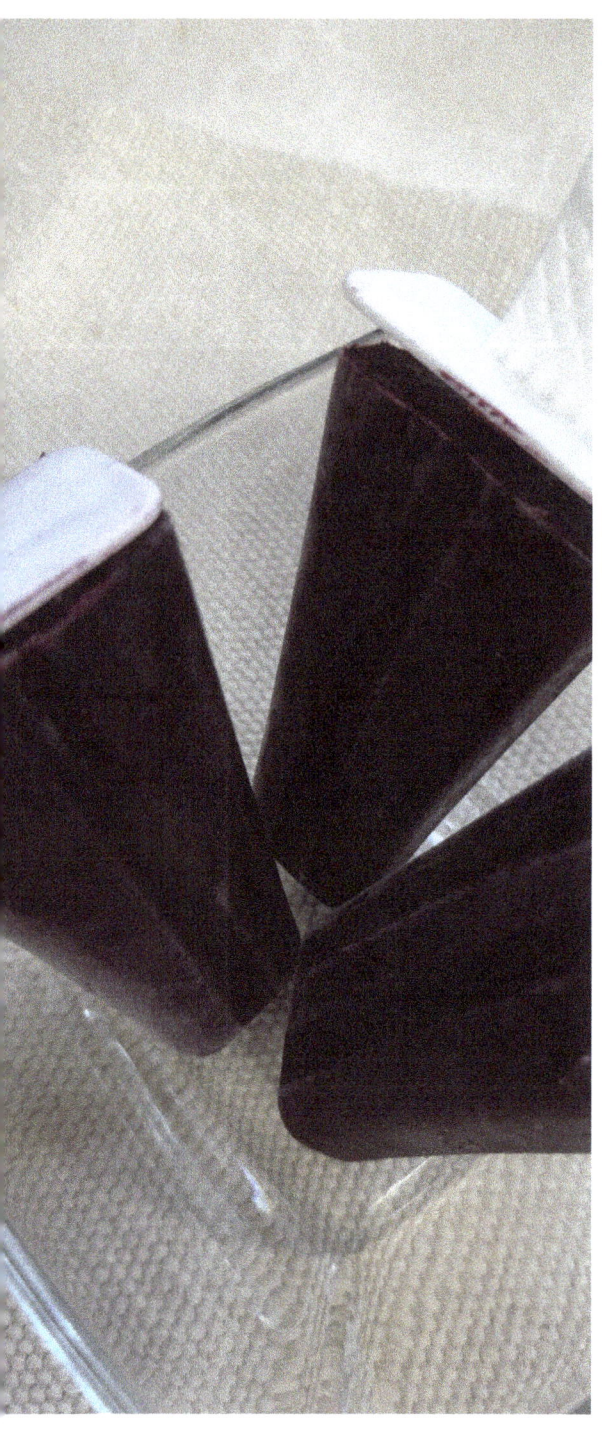

Blueberry ice cream

Ingredients:
1 cup blueberries
1 teaspoon essential rum
½ cup of coconut milk

Methods: cook the above on low heat for 15 minutes. Let it cool, then pour into the ice cream mould, place it in the freezer.

Baked pears

Ingredients:
4/5 small pears
½ lemon juice
gluten-free corn flakes
pinch of cinnamon

Methods: cut the pears in half and remove the core, place in the oven, add all the other ingredients, and bake for 20 minutes, then remove. Served with pudding or ice cream.

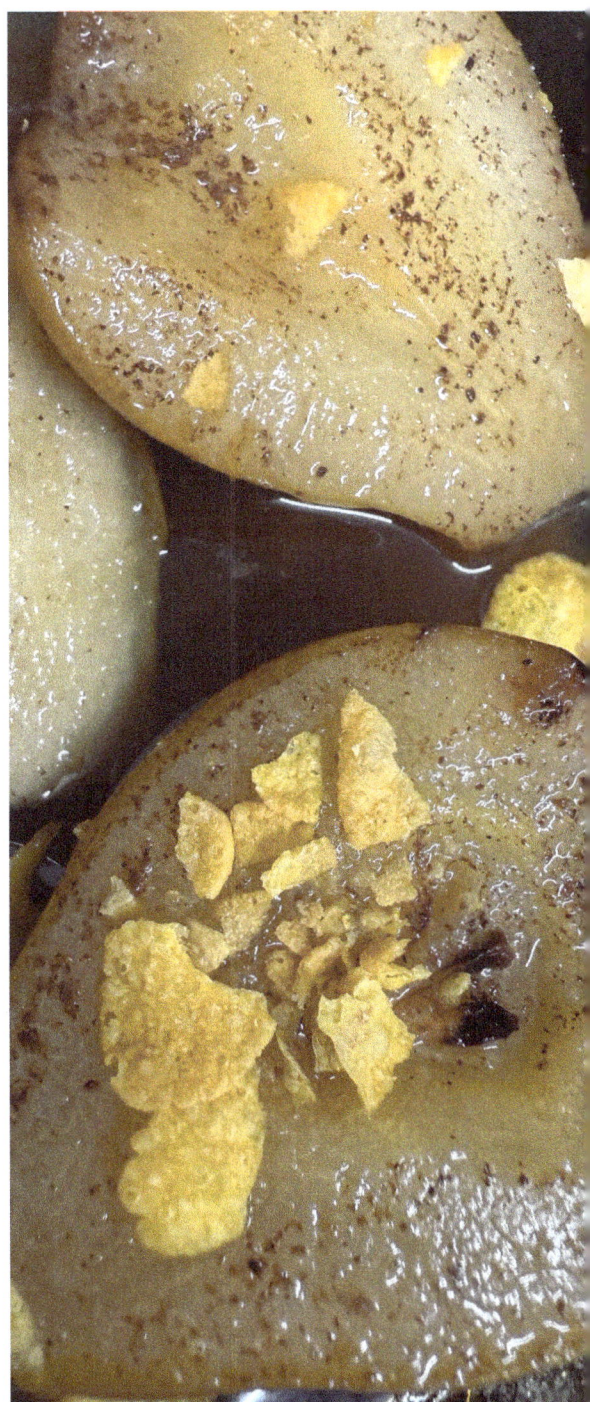

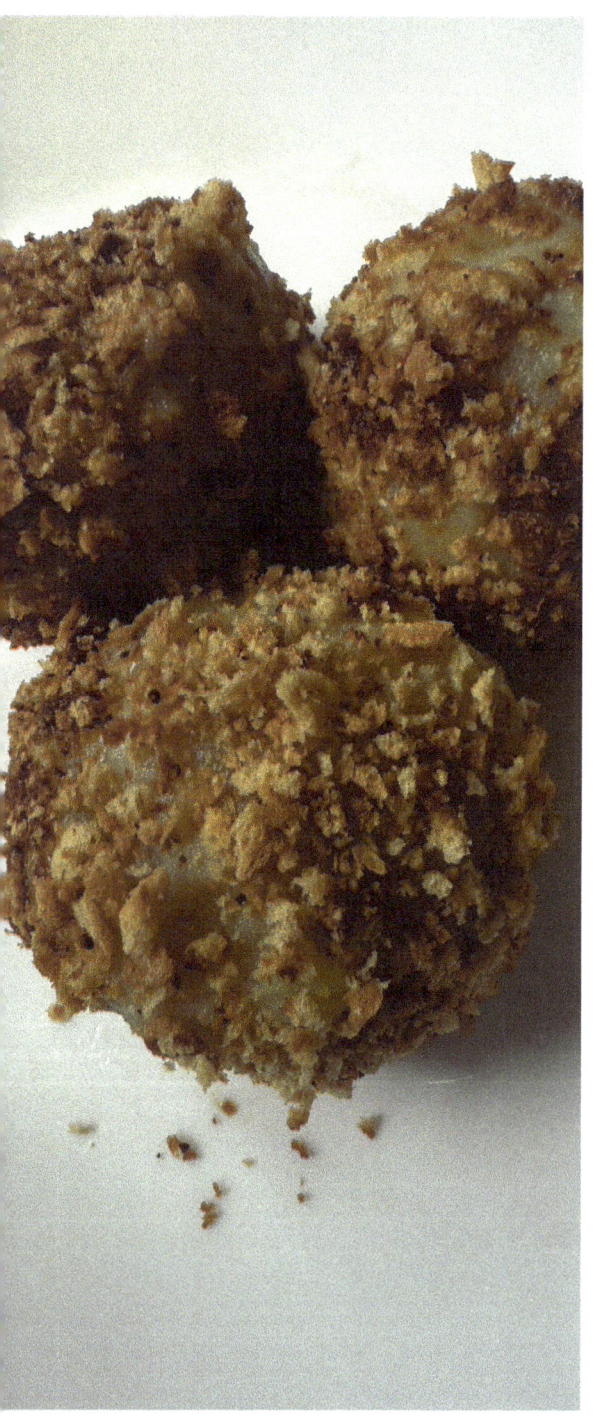

Plum dumplings

Ingredients:
2 small potatoes
250mg gluten-free flour
250ml coconut milk
250ml water
1 tablespoon olive oil
pinch of salt
8 medium plums, pitted 250mg gluten-free breadcrumbs

Methods: boil potatoes, after grating them, add the flour, water, milk, oil, and mix. Make a dough. Pinch small pieces from dough add the plum in and make a round roll. Boil them for 10minutes. Fry the breadcrumbs in a pan over low heat. Put the plums in the same pan and rolled plum dumplings in the fried breadcrumbs. Served them hot or cold.

Summary

In this book, I write about my own experience, describing a slice of my life that was honestly a challenge. It was not an easy road, and skipping down its bumpy side was rather illuminating.

I didn't choose the path; it chose me...

Unusual things happen to us in life. This happened to me a few years ago, making me realize that food not only heals, but can also make you sick.

It's almost unbelievable how tightly hidden the food culture can be within every meal. I haven't thought about how tasty I found the food from the Hungarian culture.

My mother cooked it for me from the very first moments of my life and, since then, wherever I've been around the world, I have been looking for those flavors everywhere. Food has color, taste, scent, beauty, and all of this should not be taken for granted. The food we eat serves the integrity of our body and not the other way around. Eating only the food you love without listening to your body is nothing short of arrogance.

I was stunned to realize that I should not view food as the meaning of life, but rather as a tool.

Because I don't live to eat; I eat to live (Quintilian).

In this book, I have presented you with some life-changing tips that I spent a long time researching and which aided my recovery. I am happy to share them with you.

Let's live in harmony not only with the food we eat, but with our own bodies and our environment. But how can we move on if we stumble? And what are we likely to stumble over?

How do we move on when our bodies are no longer happy with the flavors our own culture provides? Do we stumble on and ignore it, or do we do something about it?

Stress is an unavoidable part of our lives, so we need to understand how to live with it and mobilize it for our benefit, rather than letting it harm us.

Pay attention to your body and consider how you should be treating it, before it screams for help. Sometimes it is not enough simply to acquire the necessary knowledge for our recovery, without also considering how to apply it.

In order to enjoy a healthy lifestyle, we must first live in harmony with ourselves and then with those around us. Not only our food, but also our human relationships are important, and getting enough sleep is an essential part of the mental health balance.

We have to maintain our bodies in the same way as we would look after a car, checking it over every month, replacing what doesn't work and adding what is missing. Just as the car needs to pass its annual MOT, you also need to make sure you are functioning correctly in order to be able to prevent any health issues from developing. I believe it's our duty and responsibility to take care of our own body. Our unbelievable physical system is fighting for us to stay alive every single day! We must not view our body as our enemy, but as a highly developed machine that is ready to fight against the pathogens when needed.

Inspired by

Dr Bukovski, Igor: 'A természetgyógyász'.2003, Publishing House: Life and Health, Bucharest.

Giulia, Enders: 'Good'.2014 by Ullstein Buchverlage, Berlin

Dr. Julian, Melgosa: 'No stress'.2000, Publishing House: Life and Health, Bucharest.

Tess, Daly: '4 steps for a healthier you',2023, Trunsworld Publishers, London

Dr. Sarah, Brewer:'A - Z guide to Vitamins and Minerals', DrSarahBrewer.com

Rhiannon, Lambert:'The science of nutrition',2021, Penguin Random House, London

T.C. Hale: 'Kick your fat in Nuts',2012, Words to Spare, Great Britain, www. KickItInTheNuts.com

Brook, Goldner:'Goodbye Lupus Hello delicious, 2023, by Plant –Based Health Group, Houston, Texas.

Dr Broom Goldner, Goodbye autoimmune disease by, LLC Austin, Texas

Evangelical Lutheran Church in Hungary, Guide, Budapest, **Luther Kiadó**

Matt, Haig:'Reasons to stay alive, 2016, by Canongate Books Ltd, Edinburgh

www.ingramcontent.com/pod-product-compliance
Lightning Source LLC
Chambersburg PA
CBHW061225070526
44584CB00029B/3986